KETO DIET FOR WOMEN

A Complete Guide for a High-Fat Diet to Lose Weight, Gain Boundless Energy, Heal Your Body, and Regain Confidence

By

Lisa Jones

Copyright © 2019 by Lisa Jones

All rights reserved.

TABLE OF CONTENTS

Chapter 1: What Exactly Is The Ketogenic Diet?...........1

Chapter 2: Who Is The Ketogenic Diet Intended For? .27

Chapter 3: Advantages Of The Ketogenic Diet 55

Chapter 4: Cheese And A Healthy Ketogenic Meal 79

Chapter 5: Regularly Asked Questions About The Ketogenic Diet 102

CHAPTER 1
WHAT EXACTLY IS THE KETOGENIC DIET?

A Ketogenic diet is one that is very low in carbs but high in fats and is average on protein. Over the years, Ketogenic diets have been used to remedy a number of illnesses that human beings have come to face. These include; remedying weight gain as well as treating or curing ailments in human beings such as treating epilepsy among children.

The Ketogenic diet forces the human body to use its fats rather than burn its carbohydrates. Usually, the body's carbohydrates, which are found in the foods you consume, are converted into glucose. The glucose is as a result of the body burning down its carbohydrates and is usually circulated around the body. Glucose is a very important element in that it ensures the day to day functioning of your brain. However, the liver is forced to convert fats into fatty acids and ketone bodies if only very little carbohydrates are left in the food substances that you consume. These ketone bodies assume the place of the glucose in ensuring the day to day functioning of your brain. Elevated levels of ketone bodies in the human blood, a metabolic state known as ketosis, leads to a reduction of epileptic seizures. Ketosis is actually normal. It is a consequence of a low-carb diet or as a result of fasting. Ketosis provides an extra source of energy for your brain in the form of ketones.

Children or young adults suffering from epilepsy and they have tried this diet as a way to remedy their ailment have succeeded in reducing their number of epileptic seizures by half and, the success had carried on even when they opted to do away with the diet. Adults suffering from epilepsy could as well enjoy the benefits of adapting to the Ketogenic diet.

The earliest therapeutic diet (specifically for pediatric epilepsy) regulated the proteins in the human body to ensure the growth and repair of the body as well as to ensure there were sufficient calories in the body to maintain the correct height and weight of an individual. The Ketogenic diet was shaped to treat pediatric epilepsy in the year 1920 and was widely and commonly used a decade after 1920. However, with the introduction of the anticonvulsant medication, the popularity of the Ketogenic diet as a way of remedying pediatric epilepsy greatly reduced. The anticonvulsant medication was highly effective and thus, it was preferred to the Ketogenic diet.

The Ketogenic diet advocates for excluding high-carbohydrates foods or beverages such as; bread, sugar, grains, starchy vegetable, and fruits, pasta as well as beer. Instead, the Ketogenic diet advocates for high consumptions of foods or beverages that are high in fats such as; butter, cream, nuts as well as sparkling water as a beverage. The dietary fat is largely made of molecules known as triglycerides (LCTs) but the fatty acids are made up of molecules known as medium-chain triglycerides (MCTs), which are more Keto friendly. The MCT Keto diet is known to use coconut oil, which in turn is very rich in medium-chain triglycerides to ensure the provision of calories in the body. This allows room for you to choose a variety of foods to consume in that you would be bound to consume large proportions of carbohydrates and protein.

The Ketogenic diet has been studied extensively and found to be a remedy to a number of neurological disorders; brain cancer, Parkinson's disease, autism, neurotrauma, Alzheimer's disease, pain, sleep disorders, and amyotrophic lateral sclerosis.

The Ketogenic diet is beneficial in that it reduces blood sugar levels as well as insulin levels in your body. This is because the Ketogenic Diet shifts the body's metabolism to fat and ketone bodies away from carbs.

History Of The Keto Diet

The Ketogenic diet is actually a form of treatment that was established in order to improve achievement as well as omit the limitations of using fasting as a method of treating epilepsy. The use of the Ketogenic diet, as stated earlier, was more popular in the 1920s and the following decade, but the diet was abandoned after the introduction of new anticonvulsants drugs. It was proved that individuals with epilepsy could control their seizures by the use of drugs and medication; thus, rendering the Keto diet inappropriate. However, not all people find medication effective in controlling their epileptic seizures; thus, the diet has successfully found its way back in controlling epilepsy.

Before attempting to understand the introduction of the Ketogenic diet as a way of controlling epilepsy, we need to first explore the reasons why the diet was born and what was used prior to the diet.

Fasting

Fasting was used to cure epilepsy in ancient times. Physicians treated or curbed ailments such as epilepsy by simply making changes to the diet of their patients. However, the cause of epilepsy, as well as its cure, was blamed on supernatural forces, and the altering of an individual's diet was seen as ineffective. There was one case that led to the use of fasting as a way of curing epilepsy where a man was deprived of food or any drinks and ended up surviving epilepsy. Thus, the physicians of the old days would put a patient in the fasting mode until he was cured. This was to be carried out without mercy or wishes of the patient to have food or something to drink.

Despite the use of fasting as a way of remedying epilepsy being in existence as far back as the 400 BC in ancient Greece, fasting was first studied as a way of curing epilepsy in 1911 in France. About twenty patients of epilepsy of different ages were constrained to a low-calorie vegetarian, diet which was accompanied by purging as well as fasting. However, only two out of the twenty patients found success in the diet, while the remaining patients did not find success in the diet. It was found that the diet improved the patient's mental health contrary to their medication, which mostly comprised of potassium bromide that subdued the patient's mind.

It was about this time that an American advocate of physical culture, Bernarr Mcfadden, made fasting popular as he used it to restore his patient's health. During this same time, Bernarr's disciple Dr. Hugh William Conklin, an American, started treating his patients of epilepsy by recommending fasting. Dr. Hugh claimed that a patient's epilepsy was a result of a toxin that was secreted in their intestines, finding its way into their body's bloodstream, causing epileptic seizures in the end. Thus, Dr. Hugh suggested fasting that would last up to 25 days to give the toxin in the intestines a chance to disappear. He went on to treat vast numbers of patients with fasting as a way of treating epilepsy. Later on, it was found that of all the patients Dr. Hugh treated, 20% were relieved of the seizures while 50% had or experienced slight improvements.

Dr. Hugh's fasting as a way of treating epilepsy was adopted by neurologists as well. A certain Dr. McMurray in the year 1916 claimed to have successfully treated his epileptic patients by suggesting a fast period to them that was accompanied by both sugar and starch free diet in his letter to the *New York Medical Journal.*

Endocrinologist Henry Geyelin, who had experienced Dr. Hugh's use of fasting to treat epilepsy first-hand, also attempted to treat his own epileptic patients using the same method and succeeded. Continued studies in the 1920s reported the seizures would return after even after a patient had fasted in the suggested period of time.

Diet

Rollin Turner, in the year 1921, had the opportunity to review the diet and diabetes research. He concluded that the liver of a normal healthy human being who was deprived of water and food put through fasting would produce ketone bodies, acetoacetate, and hydroxybutyrate, which were soluble water compounds. This would happen if the patient fasted or adopted a low carbohydrate and a high-fat diet for a given period of time. It was Dr. Russell Wilder, of Mayo Clinic, who built on Robin's research and later came up with the *'Ketogenic diet'* which represented a diet that was used to produce elevated levels of ketones in the body through increased consumptions of fats and limited consumptions of carbohydrates. Dr. Russell hopes were to get the same results that fasting produced, but instead, he hoped to have these results in a diet that an epileptic patient could adapt to and find a remedy to the ailment for life. His usage of the diet on patients was the first time he put his diet on trial and used the diet to treat epilepsy in the year 1921.

Pediatrician Mynie Peterman is credited with creating the classic Keto diet later on. Mynie's work is what led to the introduction and maintenance of the diet. Mynie would document the positive effects of the diet, which included enhanced alertness, enhanced behavior, as well as better sleep. Mynie also documented the side effects of the diet which included vomiting and nausea, which was caused by the excess ketosis a patient would experience. However, the Keto diet found success in children. Mynie would report that a large percentage of up to 95% of the younger patients would have better control of their seizures, and 60% of the young patients would eventually become seizure-free. As time progressed, the Ketogenic diet was extensively studied in adults as well as teenagers. Reports by Clifford Barborka claimed that the diet was effective for children rather than adults, and thus, the Ketogenic diet in adults was left unstudied until the end of the century in 1999.

Anticonvulsants and the Decline of the Keto Diet

As stated earlier, the Ketogenic diet was only popular and extensively studied in the 1920s stretching to the 1930s at the time when the only anticonvulsant drugs were the sedatives bromide, which was discovered in 1857 and phenobarbital which was discovered in 1912. However, all the attention that was generated by the Keto diet was done away with in 1938 when Houston Merritt Jr., as well as Tracy Putnam, made a new discovery and discovered the drug phenytoin. It was during this time that research on cures and treatment shifted focus and focused on drugs; thus, the Keto diet's reputation slowly declined.

With the coming of drugs, neurologists had an effective way of treating vast ranges of epileptic syndromes as well as different types of seizures. A good example of these drugs was sodium valproate in the 1970s, which gave neurologists options. The use of the Keto diet as a way of treating epilepsy was restricted to more complex cases such as the Lennox-Gastaut syndrome, and thus, its usage further declined.

The MCT Diet

Introduced to you earlier in this book, the MCTs (medium-chain triglycerides) were reported to be an effective way of producing more ketone bodies in the 1960s. This was contrary to the dietary fats, which are often long-chain triglycerides, and which produced fewer ketone bodies per unit of energy. The MCTs are easily absorbed and quickly carried to the liver.

The restriction to carbohydrates that was advocated for by the Keto diet made it a problem for most parents to prepare meals that their children would find appropriate. Thus, a certain Peter Huttenlocher came up with a new Keto meal plan that consisted of more than half the meal being made from MCT oils in 1971. This new Keto meal plan allowed room for consumption of more protein as well as three times the consumption of carbohydrates compared to the previous Keto meal plan and still get the desired effects. He went on and tested this new Keto meal plan on children as well as adults who all suffered from epileptic seizures and found out that a large number of children had improved in controlling their seizures as well as their alertness, just like the previous Keto meal plan. This new Keto meal plan was found to be more appropriate to make, and thus, children could effectively adapt to the diet as a way of treating epileptic seizures. The MCT diet took the place of the Keto diet, and it became more popular in hospitals, thus leading to the decline of the Keto diet.

The Revival of the Keto diet

The Ketogenic diet found its way back in the world many years after its decline in the case of a Hollywood producer, Jim Abrahams, whose two-year-old son had suffered extensively from epilepsy in 1994. Therapies, as well as mainstreams that were applied to the young boy, could not control the epilepsy. Abrahams found about the Ketogenic diet as he went through an epilepsy guide for his son and took his son to a pediatric neurologist at *John Hopkins Hospital* who specialized in epilepsy. John Freeman put the two-year-old Charlie through the Ketogenic diet, and his health improved drastically. This encouraged Abrahams to start the Charlie Foundation to create awareness of the diet as well as raise funds to sustain the research on the diet.

Abrahams' determination to creating awareness on the Ketogenic diet paid off because, in 1998, results of research on the diet were published by the *American Epilepsy Society*. In 1997, Abrahams, who is a movie director, produced a Television movie which was titled *First Do No Harm,* which involved a young boy who was suffering from epilepsy finds treatment after adapting and maintaining the Ketogenic diet.

After these efforts, by 2007, the Ketogenic diet was being used for epilepsy treatment by over 45 countries in the world for both children and adults. Further research on the diet is still ongoing to determine how effective the diet could be on other disorders apart from epilepsy.

Types of Keto Diets

There are several types of Ketogenic diet that you could adapt and maintain. These include;

- **The Standard Ketogenic Diet (SKD):** In simple terms, this is a very low-carb diet accompanied by high-fats and average protein that is consumed by human beings. It consists of 70% to 75% fats, 20% protein and about 5% to 10% carbs. This translates to about 20 – 45 grams of carbohydrates, 40 – 65 grams of proteins, but no set limits for fats which makes up for large parts of the diet. This is because fats are what provide the calories, which constitute energy and make the diet a successful Ketogenic diet. Additionally, there is no limit to the fats because different human beings have different energy requirements. The Standard Ketogenic Diet is successful in assisting people in losing weight, improving the body's glucose as well as improving heart health.

- **Targeted Ketogenic Diet (TKD):** This type of Ketogenic Diet focuses its attention on the addition of carbs during workout sessions only. This type of Ketogenic diet is almost similar to the Standard Ketogenic Diet except for the fact that carbohydrates are all but consumed during workout sessions. This type of diet is solely based on the idea that the body will effectively and efficiently process carbohydrates consumed before or during a workout session. This is because the diet assumes that the muscles would be bound to demand more energy, which would be provided by the carbohydrates consumed and be processed quickly since the body is in an active state. This diet, in simpler terms, is a diet caught up between the Cyclical Ketogenic diet and the Standard Ketogenic Diet, which allows room for consumption of carbohydrates on the days that you would decide to work out only.

- **High-Protein Ketogenic Diet:** This type of Ketogenic Diet advocates for more protein compared to the **Standard Ketogenic Diet.** This diet consists of 35% protein, 60% fats, and 5% carbs, unlike the Standard Ketogenic Diet. Research has greatly suggested that this diet would be effective for you if you are attempting to lose weight. However, unlike other types of the Ketogenic diet, no research has been dedicated to showing if there are any side effects of adapting to the diet for elongated periods of time.

- **Recurring Ketogenic Diet (RKD):** This kind of Ketogenic Diet focuses on higher-carb re-feeds; for instance, 5 Ketogenic days and 2 high-carb days, and the cycle is repeated. This diet is also known as the carb backloading and is often intended for athletes because the diet allows their bodies to recover the glycogen lost as a result of workouts or intense sporting activities.

- **Very low carbs Ketogenic diet (VLCKD):** As stated prior, a Ketogenic diet will most likely consist of very low carbs; thus, this diet often refers to the characteristics of the Standard Ketogenic Diet.

- **The Well Formulated Ketogenic Diet:** this term is as a result of one of the leading researchers into the Ketogenic diet, Steve Phinney. As the name suggests, this diet has its fats, carbohydrates, and proteins well formulated and that it meets the standards of a Ketogenic diet. This diet is also similar to the Standard Ketogenic Diet, and this means that it creates room for your body to undergo ketosis effectively.

- **The MCT Ketogenic Diet:** The diet is also related to the Standard Ketogenic Diet only that it derives most of its fats from medium-chain triglycerides (MCTs). This diet will often use coconut oil which has high levels of MCTs. This diet has been reported to efficiently treat epilepsy because of its concept that MCTs give your body enough room to consume carbohydrates as well as proteins and still maintain your body's ketosis. This is a result of MCTs providing more ketones per gram in fat contrary to the long-chain triglycerides, which are more common in normal dietary fats. However, MCTs could lead to diarrhea as well as stomach upsets if this diet is consumed in large quantities on its own. To handle, it is wise to prepare a meal with a balance of both MCTs and fats with no MCTs. There is no evidence to prove that this diet could as well have benefits in your attempt to losing weight or if the diet could regulate your body's blood sugar.

- **The Calorie Restricted Ketogenic Diet:** This is also related to the Standard Ketogenic Diet except that its calories are only limited to a given amount only. Research has proven that Ketogenic diets could be successful whether the consumption of calories are restricted or not. The reason behind this is that the effect of consuming fats and your body being in ketosis is a way in itself that prevents you from over-eating or eating beyond your limits.

There are numerous Ketogenic diets, but the Standard Ketogenic Diet and the High-Protein Ketogenic Diets are the most studied and most recommended for health issues. The Repeated (cyclical) and Targeted Ketogenic diets remain the most practiced by athletes and bodybuilders and are more advanced than the Standard Ketogenic Diet and the High-Protein Ketogenic Diet. Visit and consult your local physician before opting to settle on any of the types of Ketogenic diets.

Implementation of the Ketogenic diet

As we have come to know, the Ketogenic diet is an effective way of treating epilepsy in children. This means that for you to attempt implementing the Ketogenic diet to your day to day life, you need the approval of your physician as well as the guidance of your physician in choosing from the types of Ketogenic diets what diet suits you best based on your reasons for wanting to practice the diet.

The implementation, as well as the maintenance of this diet, requires maximum attention from both the patient as well as the physician. The collaboration between the physician and the patient kicks off at the hospital when, during the initiation of the diet, both parties will have to attend the classes on the different mechanisms of the diet as well as the history of the diet.

Here, the physician will be your teacher and guide while you, the patient, will be the learner. The physician will take time to educate you on the history of the diet as well as take you through the different types of diet before settling down on one type of diet that you will follow strictly. The physician will also be required to explain to you the positive and negative effects of the type of Ketogenic diet that you would have found appropriate before subduing yourself to it. This will be after carefully evaluating and examining your body if you are epileptic or suggesting a given type of the Ketogenic diet if you simply want to lose weight. Afterward, the physician will also explain to you the right ways of preparing Ketogenic meals, the ingredients to use as well the ingredients to do away with.

The Ketogenic diet is implemented in five stages;

1. **The diet initiation stage:** there are two ways in which your diet could be transitioned. First, the physician will gradually increase your calorie consumption. Here, the physician will have to calculate your average consumption of calories in a day and then gradually add more calories to your meals. It could be from 1/3 of your consumption to 2/3 and finally to the amount desired or prescribed by your physician. Secondly, your physician will gradually increase your Ketogenic diet ratio, from 1:1 to 2:1 or 3:1, until the desired ratio is met. It is important to note that the Ketogenic diet will be initiated after several factors have been considered. For instance, your age, your financial status, your educational background, or your food preference. The Ketogenic diet will be initiated quicker if you are epileptic and if a quick control of seizures is desired compared to when you are using the diet to lose weight. Furthermore, fasting would be appropriate to you at the beginning of the therapy if you were

having a seizure and an effect on controlling the seizures was desired immediately. The physician will pay close attention to your body to ensure that the sugar levels are balanced so as to avoid other greater effects. Usually, your transition from a regular diet to the Ketogenic diet would last between one to two weeks, and you could either be hospitalized or you could be allowed to practice the new diet from home. This is usually to teach you the patient on the importance of implementing and strictly following the diet's requirements. However, the Classical Ketogenic diet therapy would require close supervision by a well-experienced physician, and this could mean you would have to be hospitalized in order to get the desired results. Mostly, the basic starting Ketogenic diet ratio is 2:1 to 4:1 and could take up to 2 weeks before your body completely adapts to the Ketogenic diet. The calories are usually 245-330 kj/kg body weight (62-82 kcal/kg body weight). For the case of your children, 378 kj/kg body weight (88 kcal body weight). Calories are usually calculated to 75-90% of the suggested calorie requirements depending on the age of you, the patient. However, there is a specific calorie level for each individual, and thus, it is important to measure the calorie levels every week. If you are overweight, special attention is paid by the physician in regulating your calorie consumption.

2. **The titration stage:** this is often between 1 to 6 months after the diet initiation phase. During this phase, your physician will still make adjustments to your ratio in the Ketogenic diet with the sole purpose of achieving the intended outcome.

3. **The consolidation stage:** usually, the maintenance of the Ketogenic diet as a means of treatment is roughly 2 years after the diet initiation stage. Here, your physician will assess the effect of the diet and whether your body is responding accordingly.

4. **The discontinuation stage:** this is the stage where you are no longer experiencing seizures and could last up to 2 years if you took part in the diet with the aim of treating epileptic seizures.

5. **Returning to the normal diet phase;** this is after the diet has completely acted to the desired effect and now your body is ready to make changes and accommodate the regular diet. This will usually take 3 to 6 months of

gradual transitioning to the regular diet.

Combining the Ketogenic Diet with Antiepileptic Drugs

It should be noted that not all patients will be seizure-free when the whole diet phases have been completed. Some patients may not be seizure-free by solely relying on the diet to do that but could require the combination of the Ketogenic diet with antiepileptic drugs to handle and put the seizures in check. At the start of the Ketogenic diet therapy, the administration of the antiepileptic drugs is maintained for the first three months, but gradually reduced with caution in order to accurately evaluate the effectiveness of the Ketogenic diet as well as to manage seizures as your body adapts to the diet.

Abruptly stopping on the antiepileptic drugs after adopting the Ketogenic meal plan could lead to severe effects such as; a recurrent of the seizures and you could find this uncomfortable. Thus, it is important to maintain the ingestion of the antiepileptic drugs for up to a year before considering a reduction to the dose of the drugs to allow your body a chance to adapt to life after the drugs.

Effectiveness of the Ketogenic Diet

The Ketogenic diet has been proven to minimize

seizures by up to half the number of recorded patients rendering the diet effective in its own capacity to treating epilepsy. Children suffering from refractory epilepsy have greatly benefitted from the diet and the diet has been proven a success compared to the usage of the antiepileptic drug to treat the same ailment in children. The effectiveness of the Ketogenic diet could be categorized into two stages;

- The Trial Stage
- The Outcome Stage

The Trial Stage

This is the very first time the diet was ever put into practice. Studies and research conducted during this time showed that patients showed improvements as some became seizure-free while others had their numbers of seizures reduced by half. However, the results obtained in the trial stage were biased because the results of the patients who did not find success in the diet were left out in favor of popularizing the diet and thus, results of the patients who did well were documented. In an attempt to curb this bias, the patients whose results will be judged later on are picked before the Ketogenic diet is put in action and their results are documented, whether they failed or did well in the trials.

Additionally, the kind of patients treated using the Ketogenic diet has transformed drastically over time. This is because when the diet was first put in place, it was not used to treat people who tried other forms of treatment and failed contrary to the modern ways where patients who have attempted other forms of treatment are treated using the idea and treated of their ailments.

The Outcome Stage

This is where the modern forms of the diet took root, and researches were done extensively. The *John Hopkins Hospital* in the United States published a study in 1998 that showed how effective the diet was on treating epilepsy. The study consisted of 150 children who were suffering from epilepsy and who were experiencing epileptic seizures. The children were put on the diet, and their results studied afterward. Some of these children experienced an end to seizures, while others were reported to have a reduction in seizures. Some children discontinued the diet mainly because they were significantly better. However, a small number of children discontinued the diet because it was ineffective or due to illnesses related to adopting the diet.

It is then accurate to say that the Ketogenic diet as a way of remedying epilepsy is true and very effective. This is despite the health issues that are related to the diet;

increased levels of cholesterol, or weight loss (if you are not planning on reducing weight). It is also correct to claim that the efficacy of the diet on children is also effective in adults.

Ketogenic Diet and Weight Loss

Ketogenic diets allow you to shed off excess weight without risking diseases. This diet helps you lose fat in the body as well as ensures the mass of your muscles is well preserved. The Ketogenic diet promotes weight loss through an increase in the intake of protein, which has numerous weight-loss advantages. Controlling consumptions of carbohydrates control the calorie intake, which is a key component in weight loss and burning calories as a result of the conversion of proteins and fats into carbs that run your body.

Ketogenic diets also assist in rapidly burning fats while partaking in physical exercises, rests, and other normal day to day activities, which in return help you shed off unwanted weight.

Ketogenic Diet and Diabetes

Diabetes is designated through raised levels of blood sugar, which are harmful to the heart, kidneys, nerves, and blood vessels over time. Diabetes occurs when the body is not able to yield adequate insulin or when the body becomes resilient to insulin. Type 2 diabetes is, as proved, is the most experienced type of diabetes in adults

Ketogenic diets are essential in curbing type 2 diabetes because the diet helps you shed off excess fats, which are closely associated with this site type of diabetes. The diet has been proven to assist individuals suffering from type 2 diabetes to stop using medication associated with the disease, thus ending up finding an effective treatment for the ailment.

Tips to Help You Succeed While on the Ketogenic Diet

1. **Learn to minimize your consumption of carbohydrates;** in order to achieve ketosis, the most important is doing away with high-carb diets. When you minimize your intake of carbohydrates, your body is forced to burn its fats as a way of replacing the glucose that would normally be used to energize your body. This way your body is bound to achieve ketosis.

2. **Learn to include coconut oil in your meal plan;** as we stated earlier, coconut oil is rich in MCTs, which are good in that they are

easily absorbed into the liver and be used almost immediately as a source of energy or which could as well be converted into ketones.

3. **Learn to increase your fats intake in a healthy manner;** by now you already know that consuming an increased level of healthy fats could improve the ketone levels in your body as well as help your body reach ketosis. You could also opt to choose from a variety of animal and plant fats to improve your ketone levels in the body.

4. **Learn to fast;** by fasting, you significantly improve your body's chances of reaching ketosis. You could decide to go for hours without eating. Fasting has been proven to quickly get your body into ketosis.

5. **Learn to test your ketone levels and make the right adjustments;** this is important because it will give you a chance to know if the diet is working effectively or if adjustments are needed. It is important to test your ketone levels to determine how your body is fairing.

6. **Learn to regulate your protein consumption;** in order for your body to reach ketosis, you have to ensure that your

consumption of proteins is regulated; not excessively consumed, but adequately consumed.

7. **Learn to put your body in the active state;** you could decide to engage your body in physical activities such as; jogging, swimming, hiking, playing basketball or football or going to the gym. This is important because your body ketone levels improve when your body is in an active state. You could speed up this process by fasting and working out at the same time.

CHAPTER 2
WHO IS THE KETOGENIC DIET INTENDED FOR?

As stated earlier in the first chapter, the Ketogenic diet is a remedy for a number of diseases and that in itself qualifies an individual with the ailments in question to adapt to the diet. However, the diet could also be used by other professionals in order to enhance their performances or for other reasons.

The question 'who is the Ketogenic diet intended for?' is very wide, but we are going to look at a number of people who can qualify to use this diet in their day to day lifestyles.

Ketogenic Diet and Athletes

A high fat, low carb and average protein diet could be a better option for enduring athletes. It could be essential in that the diet could help you, an athlete, perform better in the field. However, if you are a team or a sprint athlete, this diet could cause a drop in your performance as a result of adapting to it.

As you have come to see, the Ketogenic diet is not only

used for treating epilepsy or losing weight, numerous athletes have turned to this very low carb, high fats diet to boost their track performance. However, if you are an athlete and you are involved in high-intensity sporting activities such as playing basketball or football and you have adopted this diet, new research has proven that you could experience a decline in your performance.

Saint Louis University in Missouri, United States of America, conducted a research in an attempt to prove that the Ketogenic diet is not effective to high-intensity sportsmen and women. The researchers from the university opted to test the performance of a group of anaerobic athletes who were put on the Ketogenic diet and compared the results to another group who consumed a high carb diet for the same period of four days. The results indicated that the anaerobic athletes who had been on the Ketogenic diet performed poorly compared to the athletes who consumed more carbs. The research concluded that the Ketogenic diet could make a significant difference to athletes who are involved in sporting activities that are reliable on the short-burst energy. These sporting activities that use the short burst energy could include; the 100-meter sprint, the triple jump, the long jump, basketball, or soccer, and thus, this diet is not recommended for you if you are indulging in these activities. You should avoid this diet if you are an athlete that uses a lot of energy unless you have compelling reasons to use it or your physician suggested it.

However, athletes such as; long-distance cyclists, marathon runners or the 10000 meters runners could perform fairly better if they were on the Ketogenic diet compared to athletes who use short bursts of energy. This diet appears to be of benefit to athletes who have been using this diet for a good period of time claims Dr. Clifton Page, a professor of orthopedics and family medicine of the *University of Miami Miller School of Medicine.* The professor went on and claimed that the body would require a significant amount of time to stop using carbohydrates as the source of energy to using fats and called that period the 'adaptation period.' He also claimed that this period could take up to several months of sticking to the Ketogenic diet.

Dr. Page's claims were supported by Zach Bitter. Zach is a 3x Team United States of America World 100km champion and says that he consumes about 70% of fats when he is recovering from a long race or when he is working out.

This does not mean that you could consume a lot of protein since protein is what constitutes the Ketogenic diet. In fact, consuming a lot of proteins could interfere with your body's production of ketones which is what your body uses as a substitute due to the lack of glucose.

If you are an endurance athlete and you are using this diet, it may not only improve your performance, but also your health in general. Despite all this information, it is actually advisable to adapt to the Ketogenic diet if it has been designed by your physician or your nutritionist or you could also work with an individual who is more experienced in the Ketogenic diet and guide you.

Ketogenic Diet and the Military

With cases of obesity on the rise in the military, the Ketogenic diet could come in handy in the military. Obesity in the military in terms of making recruitments or maintain the fitness of the soldiers ready for service could be hugely boosted by the Ketogenic diet. You probably already know that fitness is a major element before or when you are in the military. If you ate aspiring to join the military but you are obese, the Ketogenic diet could come in handy and assist you to shed off some of that extra weight. If you are already in the military but you find yourself obese, this diet could also do the same for you. However, the most important thing is to first consult with your physician or nutritionist before starting on the diet.

A study that was conducted and which appeared on the *Military Journal* documented just how the Ketogenic diet is efficient for the military. Military participants were put on trial to reduce their weights and the diet significantly made that possible. The participants of this study reported to the physician and had their blood ketone levels checked and they were advised on their food choices ranging from drinks to foods and advised on what types of foods or drinks that could possibly maintain their body's ketosis. This proved that the Ketogenic diet could be a reliable way or means of controlling obesity, particularly the visceral adipose tissue, a type of fat in the body that is strongly linked to chronic diseases. Considering that 6 out of 10 people who aspire to join the military are dropped because of their weight, this diet comes in to help you neutralize that threat.

Ketogenic Diet and Cancer Patients

The Ketogenic diet is recommended as a way of helping cancer patients fight off cancer. This is possible because, some types of cancer do not have the ability to metabolize the ketone bodies, which are as a result of adapting to the Ketogenic diet, due to a reduced regulation of enzymes as well as mitochondrial dysfunction, which are essential for ketone utilization. Additionally, if you adopt the Ketogenic diet and you are a cancer patient, the diet attempts to target the Warburg effect which, in simplified terms, is a biochemical occurrence one in which cells of cancer greatly use glycolysis. The diet comes in at the perfect time to make that possibility much harder for the cancer cells to achieve. The diet's main purpose is to cut on the body's usage of glucose and introduce ketone bodies a situation where the cancer cells are deprived of energy while your normal body cells adapt to using the ketone bodies. To add on, the Ketogenic diet in itself regulates the insulin levels in your body that are essential in driving cancer cells to proliferate.

However, research and trials are still ongoing to determine whether the Ketogenic diet could be a remedy for a specific cancer. Most of the data obtained on the Ketogenic diet and cancer has been solely based on single case reports which limit other possibilities of the diet on cancer patients.

To conclude, for the Ketogenic diet to be used as a therapy for cancer patients, you need to first consult your physician to determine the anti-tumor effect in a clinical setting. This is because the efficacy of the diet on cancer depends on the genotype as well as the tumor entity. This is not to ignore the fact that the Ketogenic diet can be a good option for a number of cancers. In the meantime, you may sit tight and wait for the clinical trial to be complete.

Ketogenic Diet and Fertility

As we stated earlier, the Ketogenic diet could be

essentials for you considering that you are obese and looking to shed off the extra weight. Another factor to consider is that if you are obese and looking to get pregnant, your body weight could be a major challenge in getting pregnant as well as staying pregnant. Excess body fat is closely related to increased chances of suffering a miscarriage. If you are a woman and you are overweight you are probably wondering if the Ketogenic diet could assist you in shedding some extra weight and boost your fertility. The answer is yes.

You already know that the Ketogenic diet is very low in carbs and high in fats as well as average in protein and that once you adapt to it, your body gets into ketosis. This diet is essential to you for weight reduction as well as assists your body in reducing systemic inflammation which could generally reduce your fertility chances significantly.

It has been proved beyond reasonable doubt that the Ketogenic diet could help you improve your body weight and assist your body to ovulate and release an egg. This then boosts your chances of getting pregnant, given that your body is now in shape, and maintain the pregnancy. Additionally, it has been proven that the Ketogenic diet could help your body to rebalance your hormones; thus, your body could, in the future, get pregnant without the assistance of hormone-regulating drugs. If you have irregular menstruation cycles, the diet could help you to resume regular menstruation.

The Ketogenic diet is also a good friend to the men with fertility problems. Most foods are full of refined carbohydrates as well as sugars, which are all concerned with poor sperm health in men. These foods affect sperm shape and also the sperm motility. It is going to be a challenge for you to get your partner pregnant given that your sperm is good enough. After adopting the diet, results studied after trials have shown that sperm health is greatly improved, thus boosting your fertility chances.

However, using the Ketogenic diet to boost your fertility as a woman should be supervised by a nutritionist or your physician. You should only use the diet to start a new and healthy diet routine and leave it at that. This is because your body cannot be in ketosis when you are pregnant because it is advisable to eat whole foods rich in all nutrients and not limited like the Ketogenic diet. Not to forget, the Ketogenic diet increases your chances of suffering from nutrient deficiencies and you do not want your unborn baby to be nutritionally limited while in your womb. Thus, you should only use the diet to shed the extra weight and get your body in shape to get and maintain a pregnancy or get you into proper eating habits, but you should stop on the diet when you are pregnant.

Ketogenic Diet for Pregnant Women

While researchers have invested heavily in the Ketogenic diet, they have focused their attention on the diet and its treatment properties on cancer, epilepsy, and weight loss. When it comes to the properties of the diet for pregnant or aspiring to be pregnant women, researches are very rare. There have been no trials on pregnant women as this would rather increase the risks of losing the unborn baby. Generally, trials of any sort on pregnant women are discouraged.

Despite the fact that human trials on pregnant women have been discouraged, this does not mean that the research has been prohibited from other living organisms, too. According to a published study in *BMC Pregnancy & Childbirth,* constituted of pregnant mice that were put on the Ketogenic diet. The mice in the trials faced many challenges ranging from stunted growth in their offspring, larger than normal spines as well as a reduction in the size of hearts and brains. The study concluded that the application of the Ketogenic diet during pregnancy could result in changes in behavior in the offspring or organ dysfunction at large.

It should be noted that glucose which is obtained from consuming carbohydrates is the main source of energy for a given unborn baby's growth and complete development when it is still in the womb. If this is altered, the consequences could be great as the unborn baby might not fully develop in the womb and could be born with disabilities. Not only will the diet cause developmental issues to the unborn baby, but it could also be a cause of malnutrition to both the pregnant woman as well as the unborn baby and this could result in other health issues. As you already know, the diet advocates for high fats and very low carbs which means that you would have to do away with fruits and numerous vegetables to maintain ketosis. For a pregnant woman, this could be a challenge because fruits and vegetables are sources of vitamins essential for the development of unborn children since the pregnant woman would have to do away with them.

It should also be noted that adopting the diet during pregnancy could lead to significant weight loss during the pregnancy period. Unless specified by your doctor, this could be an issue. Your body's focus should be to raise and nurture a healthy baby in your womb and not worry about dieting. It could be that you are already overweight before and during the pregnancy period and wondering if weight loss is appropriate. Losing weight on the Ketogenic diet before pregnancy is actually a good thing, but shedding weight during pregnancy is not completely advisable. You should take advantage of your pregnancy and change your eating habits as well as visit the hospital to ensure that your unborn baby is developing well in your womb.

Is the Ketogenic Diet Appropriate for

Treating Gestational Diabetes During Pregnancy?

Gestational diabetes is a form of diabetes that is associated with pregnant women. It is caused by high sugar levels in the blood and could be a problem for both the mother and the unborn baby. Given your prior knowledge that the Ketogenic diet can be used to treat diabetes, you are wondering if this is the same case. The Ketogenic diet is known to remedy diabetes in non-pregnant people, but the diet is not advisable during pregnancy meaning you should probably not use it to treat diabetes.

You could opt to lower the consumption of carbohydrates in order to regulate your body's sugar levels while at the same time improving your consumption of vegetables and protein. You could also opt to eat small portions of food but eat regular meals throughout the day. This is another way of regulating your body's sugar levels without going into ketosis. By doing away with processed carbohydrates in junk foods and instead consuming more nuts, seeds or vegetables should be enough to maintain your blood sugar levels. Consult with your doctor regularly to ensure that gestational diabetes is in check.

What Is the Appropriate Diet for Pregnant

Women?

Now that the Ketogenic diet is off the table, you are probably wondering what diet to stick to. The very first thing you need to consider is that you have enough calories in your diet to ensure maximum energy for your unborn baby's development. This could possibly mean that your diet should consist of;

- **Non-starchy vegetables:** for example; kales, zucchini, green beans, spinach could all be viable options because the folate that is contained in them will greatly improve your unborn baby's nervous system as well as the fiber, they contain could be vital to keeping your baby regular.

- **Eggs:** eggs contain chlorine in them which is essential for the development of your placenta as well as important for the development of the baby's brain.

- **Red meat:** this will provide your unborn baby with iron as well as regulate your body's temperatures making it a conducive place in your body for your baby to develop.

- **Seafood (fatty):** if you can access seafood then that is great for you and your unborn baby.

Fish such as sardines or salmon could be a wise decision.

Eat healthy so that you ensure your baby is born healthy, fully developed, and fine. Consult with your nutritionist on the best foods for you and your unborn baby and get back to the Ketogenic diet when your physician deems it possible to resume.

Foods, Snacks, And Beverages That Constitute The Ketogenic Diet

Foods That Constitute the Ketogenic Diets

With the popularity of the Ketogenic diet on the rise, the need to understand the right type of foods to eat has now become a thing. All the foods you consume should be low in carbohydrates, moderate on proteins, but high in fats. You have already explored and hopefully understood the importance of this diet in the first chapter. You already know that the diet is used for treating epilepsy and diabetes as well as regulating your weight gain. Take a closer look at these foods that you could consume while on the diet;

- **Low-carb vegetables:** such as onions, pepper, green vegetables are low in carbs as well as calories, but at the same time, they are high in vitamins, specifically vitamin C, and other minerals. However, be careful not to consume vegetables with a lot of starch such as potatoes or yams because these vegetables could remove your body from ketosis. Antioxidants are also present in vegetables and are essential in protecting you radical which may cause damages to your body's cells.

- **Nuts and seeds:** almonds, sesame seeds, pistachios, macadamia nuts, cashew nuts, pecans, pumpkin seeds, chia seeds, walnuts are all low in carbohydrates, but high in fats. Making a habit of eating seeds is associated with the reduction of the risk of heart-related diseases. Seeds are rich in fiber as well which acts as an anti-aging agent.

- **Butter and cream:** both butter and cream contain low levels of carbs. Despite the notion surrounding butter and cream that it may cause heart diseases, extensive studies on these two have shown that moderate consumption could essential in reducing your chances of heart attacks or even strokes. Butter and cream also promote weight loss making them Keto-friendly.

- **Poultry and Meat:** steak, ham, bacon, turkey, sausage are all considered to be

Ketogenic friendly. Meat, as well as poultry, is rich in potassium, zinc, and vitamin C. No carbs are present which makes the meal Keto-friendly and they also contain proteins that help in preserving your muscles when you opt to stick to the Ketogenic diet.

- **Cheese:** that which is not processed is recommended. Cheese is a very nutritious meal. There are several types of cheese, but the most common thing amongst all of them is the fact they are very high in fat and very low in carbs which is what a Ketogenic meal should have. Cheese is rich in conjugated linoleic acid which is a fat that responsible for fat loss in the body. Cheese is also responsible for the reduction of muscle mass as a result of aging. Generally, cheese contains calcium, fatty acids, and proteins, which are important in your body when ingested.

- **Appropriate oils:** oils such as coconut oil or avocado oil as well as olive oil are all Keto-friendly. Coconut oil to be specific has MCTs, which are easily absorbed by the liver and help in the formation of ketone bodies and could as well be used as an instant energy source. It has been studied and proven that coconut oil increases ketone bodies in people suffering from Alzheimer's disease who have adopted the Ketogenic diet meal plan. Another benefit of oil is that it helps overweight people to lose weight. Olive oil, on the other hand, contains antioxidants that are important in ensuring a healthy heart.

- **Seafood:** as we stated earlier, fish such as salmon and sardines are rich in vitamin B, selenium, and potassium. These fish are free of carbohydrates making them Keto-friendly in the process. A steady consumption of these fish is closely associated with the reduction of the risk of contracting heart diseases and improves mental health. Shellfish could also be a good example of Keto-friendly seafood.

- **Avocado:** they contain lots of potassium in them which is a very important element in your body as you attempt to transition into the Ketogenic diet. Avocados also play a role in regulating the cholesterol in your body as well as triglycerides levels. They also improve markers related to the heart.

- **Eggs:** are Keto-friendly in that they contain a very low amount of carbs, but moderate levels of proteins. Egg yolks are rich in healthy cholesterol which could be essential in reducing your chances of contracting heart diseases. Eggs are also rich in other nutrients which could be important in ensuring your eyes are well maintained.

- **Berries:** unlike most fruits, berries are very low in carbs, but rich in fiber making them Keto-friendly. Berries contain antioxidants that are responsible for the reduction of inflammation and protect your heart from contracting heart diseases.

- **The Shirataki noodles:** the word is derived from the Japanese word 'shirataki,' which translates to 'white waterfalls,' which again describes the physical appearance of the noodles. They are low in carbs which makes them Keto-friendly. They are rich in fiber and have unique qualities that slow down the movement of foods in your intestine giving your body a chance to absorb nutrients effectively. This unique quality comes in handy when you are attempting to lose weight or manage diabetes. They also leave you with the effect of fullness.

Healthy Ketogenic Snacks

Almost all the snacks that first come to mind are high in carbs and thus, are not Keto-friendly. This could be very frustrating if you have just started on the diet and you find yourself hungry in between meals and the need to replenish yourself is overwhelming. Worry not! This book will certainly cater to that need. These are some of the snacks that you could consume to replenish your body in the case that you get hungry between meals for a number of reasons and you would need to feed again. The following snacks are all Keto-friendly;

- Fatty meat and fish (meatball slides)
- Strawberries and cream
- Guacamole with vegetable sticks
- Low carbohydrates milkshake with almond milk, nutritional berries, and cocoa which is powder form
- Cheese
- Cheese with olives
- Boiled eggs
- Small portions of leftover meals
- Dark chocolate (90%)
- Ketogenic smoothies
- Fermented vegetables including fermented cabbage, cauliflower, green beans, beets,

carrots, or cucumbers.

- Buffalo cauliflower bites served with blue cheese and carrot sticks.
- Coconut yogurt as an alternative for regular or traditional yogurt.
- Ground flax seeds accompanied by cheese.
- Mix nuts including almonds, pecans, Brazil nuts, cashew, walnuts, and pistachios.
- Avocado usage in the place of mayonnaise while consuming the egg salad.
- Sushi rolls that support the Ketogenic diet.
- Mix mayonnaise with cooked salmon and have a salad that is Keto friendly.

Ketogenic beverages

Foods high in carbs are not recommended the Ketogenic Diet. This also applies to drinks and beverages. Drinks that have high levels of carbs should be avoided. Soda, coffee drinks or iced tea are some of the drinks that you should abstain from. In simpler terms, all drinks that you intend to ingest must be in line with the requirements of the Ketogenic diet. Furthermore, avoid all sugar-sweetened drinks, fruit juice included because they have sugar which constitutes the consumption of carbs. Traces of carbs are also found in dairy milk omitting milk as Keto-friendly. In the meantime, water, green tea (unsweetened), sparkling water (a good replacement for soda once you consider ditching soda and challenge), unsweetened coffee, bone broth, and nut milk are Keto-friendly drinks you could opt to use.

What to Avoid

Ketogenic diets, as stated earlier in this book, support foods with low-carbs meaning any foods that have high levels of carbs should be avoided.

- **All sugary foods:** fruit juice, candy, soda, cake, honey or maple syrup, all sugar-sweetened products, sports drinks

- **Unhealthy fats:** processed vegetable oil, mayonnaise,

- **Alcohol:** alcohol constitute of high-carb content and thus, should be avoided

- **Roots vegetables and tubers:** root vegetables, potato chips, sweet potatoes, carrots, French fries, yams, etc.

- **Beans or legumes:** pears, lentils, chickpeas

- **Most fruits:** with the exception of a limited

portion of strawberries, all fruits should be avoided including mangoes, bananas, oranges, apples, etc.

- **Grains and all grain-based foods:** rice, pasta, cereals, wheat, corn, granola, cereal, etc.

The most important thing to do on the Keto diet is to personalize the diet to your lifestyle. Once you have adjusted the diet to your preference or goals in life, it becomes more enjoyable and easier to achieve as well as maintain the diet for your specific duration of time.

Supplements for the Ketogenic Diet

Since the Ketogenic diet limits food options, the idea to supplement the diet with specific nutrients is not so bad after all. Not to forget that some of these supplements will help your body to reduce the negative effects of the diet such as Ketogenic flu and even boost your athletic performance when you are on the diet. Usually, the Ketogenic diet does not require supplements, but here are supplements that come in handy. These include:

- **Minerals:** The addition of salt or other minerals is essential especially when you are starting out as a result of a shift in water and mineral balance. Magnesium consumption would be important in that boosts your energy levels, improves your immune system and regulates blood sugar levels and also because when on the Ketogenic diet, it could be a problem to consume foods rich in magnesium like beans or fruits. Supplementing with magnesium could help minimize the difficulty in sleeping and muscle cramps.

- **Caffeine:** Caffeine enhances energy or performance and also enhances fat loss in the human body. If you are an athlete and your body is attempting to transition to the Ketogenic diet, supplementing your diet with caffeine could be a good idea.

- **Exogenous ketones:** This is a supplement that assists in raising ketone levels in human blood. They are ketones that are supplied to your body by external means. Exogenous ketones as supplements are beneficial in that they help to boost your athletic performance and decrease your food appetite while on the Ketogenic diet.

- **MCT Oil:** This supplement is usually added to yogurts or other drinks and like **exogenous ketones,** it assists in raising ketone levels in the human blood. Coconut oil is a good example. Supplementing with MCT oils is essential in that it assists you in increasing your fat intake and help your body to stay on ketosis. You could add MCTs to smoothies or even ingest them directly by measure of a spoon.

- **Creatine:** This is an essential supplement for you if you are an exercising person and helps you maintain the Ketogenic Diet. It also has several health benefits and improves your performance.

- **Whey:** A little consumption of this supplement ensures your protein intake levels are maintained and can be added to yogurts.

- **Vitamins:** supplementing with Vitamin D could be important because the vitamin helps your body to boost its immune system, lowering inflammation, enhancing bone growth as well as regulating the growth of cells in your body. Ensure you consult your doctor before opting to supplement your diet with Vitamin D.

The reason why supplements for the Ketogenic diet are considered important is simply because they make the transition from your regular food to the Ketogenic diet easier. They help reduce the symptoms that come with adopting the diet such the Keto flu. Ingesting these supplements could provide your body with nutrients and give your body room to blossom while on the Ketogenic diet.

Guidelines for Ingesting out on a Ketogenic Diet

You could find yourself working late in the office or stuck in traffic for long periods of time and you could start to wonder if you could get the time to prepare yourself a Ketogenic meal. You may not have the time to prepare yourself that meal and end up being forced to dine in a restaurant. Worry not! These tips will guide you on what to eat in diners or restaurants and still maintain your Ketogenic diet meal plan.

It is actually very easy to make most of the meals served in restaurants Keto-friendly when you are dining out. You could combine a few foods and end up eating a meal that is Keto friendly.

You could eat egg-based meals in the restaurant such as omelet or bacon which support the Ketogenic Diet and still maintain your body on ketosis perfectly well.

Replacing the high-carb foods with lots of vegetables is another good option or you could decide to order for the bun-less burger and replace the fries with green vegetables to go with cheese and avocado.

As for dessert, you could opt to order berries with cream or order for a mixed cheese board.

It is recommended that while dining out, you should serve a meal with either meat, fish, or any egg-based dish as well as ingest vegetables instead of high-carb foods and having cheese for dessert. It takes time before you can fully master how to dine out and still be on your Keto meal plan. This means you should be easy on yourself and learn as time goes by.

A Sample Meal Plan for the Ketogenic Diet for 7 Days

Day 1

Breakfast: Ketogenic milkshake, vegetables omelet

Snack: sunflower seeds

Lunch: goat cheese, nuts, salsa, guacamole

Snack: celery

Dinner: Salmon with asparagus cooked in butter

Day 2

Breakfast: goat cheese omelet, hard-boiled eggs

Snack: sliced cheese

Lunch: tuna salad, almond milk, feta cheese

Snack: roast beef

Dinner: roasted chicken, broccoli, and salad

Day 3

Breakfast: bacon, scrambled eggs, tomatoes

Snack: plain

Lunch: spinach salad, peanut butter, cocoa powder, grilled salmon

Snack: smoothie from almond milk

Dinner: red cabbage, meatballs, cheddar cheese

Day 4

Breakfast: omelet, peppers, onion, protein powder, greens

Snack: a small amount of berries

Lunch: sashimi, shrimp salad, avocado

Snack: macadamia nuts

Dinner: Whitefish, spinach made with coconut oil

Day 5

Breakfast: fried eggs, mushroom

Snack: hard-boiled eggs

Lunch: a handful of nuts

Snack: celery sticks

Dinner: broccoli, peppers, peanut sauce, bun-less burger

Day 6

Breakfast: baked eggs, vegetables

Snack: kale chips

Lunch: salad, beef

Snack: pork

Dinner: vegetables, chicken, cream cheese

Day 7

Breakfast: fried eggs, stevia, peanut butter

Snack: sliced cheese

Lunch: guacamole, salsa, avocado

Snack: turkey

Dinner: salad, steak, eggs

It is always a good idea to attempt to revolve around vegetables and meat. This is because both have nutrients that are beneficial for your health over the course of your

Ketogenic Diet plan.

How to Motivate Yourself in Order to Maintain a Healthy Ketogenic Diet

The best way to motivate yourself while on the diet is simply by reminding yourself why you decided to adopt the diet in the first place. If your sole purpose is losing weight, remind yourself of all the goodness that could come with the shedding of that extra weight. Remind yourself that by losing weight, you could stand a better chance of getting pregnant, if you are a woman, as well as staying pregnant. If you are a man, remind yourself that you could boost your chances of impregnating your partner if you stick to the diet and shed off that extra weight.

If your dream is to join the military, remind yourself that sticking to the diet could be the first step to getting you closer to your dreams as you shed off that extra weight. If you are on the diet as a way to treat epilepsy or to manage your cancer, remind yourself of all the goodness of enjoying a healthy body and stick to the diet.

The bottom line is, each time you feel the road of maintaining the diet is getting tougher and tougher, learn to surge on until you achieve your set targets. The best person to motivate you while on the diet is yourself!

CHAPTER 3
ADVANTAGES OF THE KETOGENIC DIET

The Keto diet has been widely used to treating a number of notable diseases and ailments. Adapting to the diet also comes with numerous advantages. In this book, we will look at the scientific advantages of the diet to your body.

Health Benefits Of Ketogenic Diets
Loss And Maintenance Of Weight

Ketogenic diets allow you to rapidly shed off extra weight without risking diseases. The Ketogenic diet restricts the intake of carbohydrates which forces your body into ketosis and thus, a reduction of body fats. This diet not only helps you in losing fat, but also ensures the mass of the muscles is well preserved. Ketogenic diets promote weight loss through an increase in intake of protein which has numerous weight-loss advantages. The diet regulates the consumption of carbohydrates which is a key component in weight loss and burning calories as a result of the conversion of proteins and fats into ketone bodies that run your body. The diet also assists in burning fats rapidly while taking part in physical exercises, during rests and other normal day to day activities.

Control of Glucose in the Body

Another advantage of adopting the diet is that it has the ability to lower and regulate your blood sugar levels. Carbohydrates are responsible for the rise of blood sugar levels in your blood and thus, that threat is eliminated once you start on the Ketogenic diet. The Ketogenic diet is known for its ability to reduce *HbA1c* – a known measure of your blood glucose control. This measure is greatly reduced by the diet of people suffering from type 2 diabetes.

The diet is also effective to the other types of diabetes such as type 1 diabetes or LADA and thus, the diet should as well regulate the glucose in your blood. It is important to note that if the diet is maintained, the chances of regulating your blood's glucose over time could help in reducing the risk of any other health complications from occurring.

A Reduction in Reliance on Medication- Related to Diabetes

As you have already been aware of the ability of the

diet to reduce your blood sugar levels, the diet also offers a chance to patients suffering from type 2 diabetes to reduce their reliance on medication. The diet, after a good while of sticking to it, will pay your efforts as you will be able to do away with the medication related to type 2 diabetes, a study found. You could completely come off your medication or the diet could help reduce your dosage. However, consult with your doctor first before doing away with the mediation.

Control of High Blood Pressure

Numerous people in the world today are living and surviving with high blood pressure. With high blood pressure, your body becomes prone to a number of ailments, for example, heart-related diseases, kidney-related disease or even stroke. The Ketogenic diet helps you in reducing the risk of all these diseases because the diet decreases your body's blood pressure levels if you are overweight or suffering from type 2 diabetes.

An Improved Mental Performance

The diet will greatly improve your ability to remember and recall as well as improve your ability to focus. Ingestion of foods such as salmon, which are Keto-friendly could possibly boost your mood as well as your learning abilities in the classroom setting. The diet could also help enhance your long-term memory.

Restoration of Insulin Sensitivity

The Ketogenic diet is known for removing the cause of insulin resistance in your body as a consequence of elevated levels of insulin in your body. The diet cuts on the ingestion of carbohydrates which is what leads to elevated levels of insulin in the body. With a reduction of insulin level in your body, the chances of burning fat in your body increases. This is because elevated levels of insulin interfere with the breaking down of fats.

Improved Cholesterol Levels

The Ketogenic diet is a great agent in ensuring that your cholesterol levels in your blood are regulated. However, it is recommended to let your doctor of physician put you on the Keto diet if you intend to regulate your body's cholesterol levels. This is because this topic on cholesterol is complicated and would definitely require qualified personnel to handle.

Satiety

The diet is also known for its ability to have a positive effect on your appetite. The moment your body succeeds in getting into Ketosis, it becomes more comfortable with burning fats which could in turn force your body to stop craving for food and thus, improving your chances of doing away with overeating. In the long end, you would most likely succeed in losing weight.

Benefits to Individuals with Diabetes

Diabetes is a result of raised levels of blood sugar which over time are harmful to the heart, kidneys, nerves, and blood vessels. Diabetes manifests when the body is not in a position to produce adequate insulin and if your body becomes tough to insulin. The diet comes in and eliminates this possibility. Ketogenic diets are essential in curbing type 2 diabetes, which is the most experienced type of diabetes among adults because the diet helps you shed extra fat which is associated with this site type of diabetes. As a result of adapting to the diet for long periods of time, you could stand a chance of coming off your medication.

Other Benefits of Ketogenic Diets

Studies conducted have shown how the Ketogenic diet has an advantage over a number of health conditions that human beings suffer from.

- **Brain injuries:** The Ketogenic diet could minimize concussions and help your body in recovering after a brain injury.

- **Cancer:** The diet reduces the growth of tumors in your body and is applied in the medical field to treat several types of cancer at large.

- **Alzheimer's disease:** The Ketogenic diet helps in regulating the symptoms of Alzheimer's disease and also slows down its progress in the body.

- **Parkinson's disease:** the diet helps in improving the symptoms of Parkinson's disease and allows you a chance to get treated for it.

- **Heart diseases:** The Ketogenic diet improves your blood sugar levels as well as your blood pressure, which are related to heart diseases.

- **Acne:** The Ketogenic diet emphasizes the consumption of low insulin and less sugar, which in turn control acne.

Challenges Associated with the Ketogenic Diet and How to Handle Them

Despite the fact that the Ketogenic diet has numerous

advantages such as; controlling weight gain, improving cholesterol levels, controlling glucose in the body, controlling high blood pressure, or remedying epileptic seizures, it has its side effects as well. As a result of adapting to the diet, there could be results in side effects to your body as it attempts to adapt to the diet. This attempt is what is known as Keto flu and is normally experienced just a few times after you have kick starts on the Keto diet.

The Ketogenic flu is responsible for nausea, sleep deprivation, poor mental function, and exaggerated hunger within short periods of time, reduced energy levels and at other times, a decrease in energy during working out exercises. One possible way of handling the Keto flu is regulating on low-carb diets for the first few days of adapting the diet and in the end, this will teach your body to burn more fat. This is because the Ketogenic diet does not include the consumption of carbs, but instead advocates for the burning of fats into ketone bodies, which in turn take the place of glucose in your body.

The Ketogenic diet is also responsible for **altering your body's water as well as mineral** balance in your body. This is why the use of supplements, such as the addition of salt in meals or the consumption of MCTs is recommended. It is recommended to eat until you are full for the first few days of adapting to the diet because it could cause weight-loss unintentionally. The diet could also lead to a **loss of salts in your body**. As your body tries to move into ketosis, you could experience a loss of salts as well as fluids in an attempt to maintain the ketosis. Keeping yourself hydrated at all times could be very important in handling this challenge. Ensuring that you supplement the lost salts will guarantee that you will not experience headaches or wooziness. You could make salt additions directly in your food or by consuming bone broths.

The diet could also **make changes to your bowels**. A result of adapting the Ketogenic diet is that you could suffer from constipation. Constipation is majorly due to a change in your diet, thus forcing your body's gut bacteria to adapt to the new meal plan and how to handle new foods of new quantities of foods. However, a change in your vowel behavior will pass over time as your body will finally make the required adjustments. You as well consume foods rich in fiber to compensate for lack of fiber in the Ketogenic diet. You could also opt to drink a lot of water as a way of remedying your constipation.

The **composition of blood in your body is also altered** as a result of a change in dietary. Your blood may experience changes particularly a rise in the levels of lipids and cholesterol which may be higher than the normal levels. If these changes are intense and your health becomes a concern, you could make a slight change to your diet. For instance, you could lower the Ketogenic ratio and reduce the amounts of fats to carbohydrates and protein in your diet.

Adapting to the diet could also **lead to leg cramps.** These cramps could be cordial in nature. However, they could become a bother with time. They are mainly caused by adapting to the Ketogenic diet and a reduction of salts is experienced. Keeping yourself hydrated and supplementing the lost salts could be enough to take care of this challenge.

The Ketogenic diet could also **lead to bad breath.** This condition is often referred to as the Keto-breath and is mostly experienced when your body is entering Ketosis. Ketone bodies could be released in your breath, or your urine or even your sweat. This, however, is usually temporary and just as leg cramps will disappear over time. You could opt to brush your teeth or use sugar-free mint gums.

Long-term adaptations to the Ketogenic diet could also come with adverse effects. Kidney stones could be a complication for you. However, kidney stones are treatable and that means you could continue sticking to the Ketogenic Diet plan.

Stunted growth in children as a result of lowered levels of insulin could also be a major challenge for you.

This is because insulin is credited for the growth of a child and it is lowered when you start adapting to the Ketogenic diet. It is advisable that children should practice the Ketogenic diet for short periods of time to avoid stunted growth or the usage of supplements of vitamins and minerals could be applied. **Women may also suffer from amenorrhea** and this may disrupt and cause changes to their menstrual cycle.

Finally, it is important to consult your doctor before starting on the Ketogenic diet so as to address all these challenges and learn more about them.

Myths and Misconceptions Concerning the Keto Diet

Myths and misconceptions are simply false or wrong ideas or concepts that people tend to have and use them. If you have decided to give the Ketogenic diet a go, these myths and misconceptions could make the whole process a challenge or increase the chance that you will not attempt the diet or even lead you to health risks if you opted to believe them. It is important to note that approaching the decision to try the diet with adequate knowledge on all the positives, negatives as well as myths and misconceptions could set you up for success.

Take a look at these myths and misconceptions

prepared for you;

The Keto Diet Allows You to Eat as Much Butter as You Want

Despite the fact that the Ketogenic diet is a diet that is rich in fats, it does not mean that you could eat as much butter as you would prefer. It is actually very easy to convince yourself that you are doing the right thing but realizing that the diet does not allow you to eat all sorts of fats is very important. The healthiest way to regulate your fat consumption is by limiting your consumption of saturated fats and improving on your intake of unsaturated fats such as olive oil or avocados, but in moderation. This myth could mislead you into overfeeding on fats and risk other complications as a result of too much fat.

Reality; *the Ketogenic diet advocates for the consumption of unsaturated fats in your diet rather than just any fats.*

You Could Go on or off the Ketogenic Diet and Still Lose Weight

Out of curiosity, most people would adopt the diet with the hope of shedding off extra weight without consulting with their physicians or doctors. As a result, they could end up starting the Ketogenic diet for one day and regularly switch to the regular diet and still expect to shed off the extra weight. For you to achieve and maintain the state of ketosis, you would be required to stick solely to the Ketogenic diet. This is because switching to the regular diet removes your body from ketosis and your body goes back to burning carbohydrates instead of fats, thus shedding that extra weight becomes a problem. The only way you are going to benefit from the diet is if you strictly maintain your eating habits in line with the diet

Reality; *shifting your attention away from the diet could possibly lead you to gain more weight rather than shed it.*

The Ketogenic Diet Is Best for Weight Loss

Just because someone you know started and benefitted from the diet does not mean the diet would do the same for you. Just because a friend of yours lost weight while on the diet does not guarantee that the diet could do the same for you. Or rather given that everyone around you is trying the diet does not mean that you should try it as well. You should be in a position to know that the only way you could shed off that extra weight is you were consistent. It is afterward that you could decide to adopt the diet and not simply because everyone around you is trying it. You should be in a position to know that there are other ways to lose weight as well as other diets to do the same. Keep an open mind and pick on a way or a diet that would best suit all your needs.

Reality; *actually, there are other diets that could be used to shed weight as well as other ways to shed weight as well.*

One Person's Ketogenic Diet Meal Plan Could Work for Everyone

It is very easy to assume that another person's Ketogenic meal plan could also work for you. You should be able to understand that another person's body needs and requirements are different to your body's needs and requirements. Their intake of carbohydrates is very different from yours and so are their dietary needs different from yours. This is why it is not advisable to jump into someone else's Ketogenic diet, but instead, it is wise to visit your doctor or physician or nutritionist to get your own dietary needs evaluated and properly met in your own meal plan.

Reality; *someone else's Ketogenic meal plan is unique only to them and getting your own Ketogenic meal plan is wise.*

Going into Ketosis Is Equal to Going into

Ketoacidosis

Ketosis is a state where your body learns to burn fats rather than the preferred carbohydrates for energy. During ketosis, your body converts fats into ketone bodies which take the place of glucose from carbohydrates and become your body's source of energy. Confusing ketosis with ketoacidosis, which is a life-threatening complication resulting from diabetes, could be very lethal. This is because you could relax and assume that just because you adopted the Ketogenic diet that your body is in ketosis. It is advisable to visit your doctor if you feel adverse changes to your body rather than assuming other things.

Reality; *you could lose your life simply by ignoring changes to your body and making your own diagnosis and administering self-treatment could be fatal.*

You Cannot Eat Fruits While on the Keto Diet

It is true that fruits and vegetables are great sources of carbohydrates and that the only things that could be free from carbohydrates are oils or meat. It is easy to believe that you should not eat fruits while on the Ketogenic diet, but the truth is that there are fruits and vegetables that are

Keto-friendly. Fruits such as berries are low in carbs and that makes them Keto-friendly, as well as zucchini or broccoli, which are low carb vegetables that you could ingest. This is why it is important to visit your doctor or nutritionist to get your meal plan in line and one which will cater to all your needs.

Reality; *you need to consult with your physician before ruling out foods on the diet.*

Mistakes Made on the Ketogenic Diet and How to Overcome Them

At this point, you already know that the Ketogenic diet strongly advocates for a very low carb and a high-fat diet. However, just because you gave up on your bread, sweats or even pasta does not mean that you are now following a Ketogenic diet. If you think you have started the Ketogenic diet but you are not seeing any changes to your body or experiencing anything to indicate that your body is in ketosis could mean that you have fallen to these few mistakes;

- **You are not consuming the right fats;** eating fats is one thing, but eating the correct fats is another thing. There is a high chance that your body is not on ketosis even if you have been on the diet for months because of ingesting the wrong fats. You should know that not all fats are made the same and given that the Ketogenic diet advocates for the consumption of fats mean you should consume the right fats. These may include; olive oil, avocado oils, coconut oil or animal fat. You should also avoid these fats in your diet; canola oil, margarine, processed vegetable oils or grapeseed oil.

- **You are consuming a lot of anti-Ketogenic snacks;** as we stated earlier in this book, there are correct snacks that support the Ketogenic diet. If you are correctly following the Ketogenic diet and your body is on ketosis, there is a high chance that you will not crave for snacks. This does not mean however that you cannot snack once in a while. Snacking correctly should be okay, but snacking on high carb foods could remove your body on ketosis as well as elevate your body's blood sugar levels. The urge to snack could mean that your Ketogenic meal plan has not met your body's nutritional needs. This is why it is important to seek the guidance of your doctor or physician.

- **You are not having enough sleep;** lack of enough sleep could make it almost impossible to repair your body for effective functioning. A study has proved that lack of sleep could lead to increased cravings for sugary foods and this could undo your body if it is in ketosis. For your body to perform and function normally, it is advisable to sleep for about 7 to 8 hours so that your body gets enough time to repair and function normally.

- **Worrying too much;** it is normal for you to worry about yourself, but the difference comes in when you decide to act on your worries. If you adopted the Ketogenic meal plan with the intention of losing weight, it is normal to lose weight on the first few days of the diet but retain some water once your body has adapted to the diet. This could mean that your weight will probably remain stagnant for a while. Constantly checking your weight over the day and worrying too much could discourage you from continuing with the diet.

- **Consuming inadequate sodium;** when your body is already adapted to the Ketogenic diet and is now fully running on ketones, sodium is more likely to be lost during excretion together with water. Not supplementing sodium could lead to the contraction of Ketogenic flu. The easiest way to curb this is by adding salt to your meals as well as drink lots of water.

Success Stories of Women Already Practicing the Keto Diet

At times, the best way to motivate yourself into achieving your set goals or targets is simply by listening to people who are already ahead of you in your journey and learning from them. This is important because by listening to them, you get a chance to learn of their challenges and be able to keep an open mind into anticipating your own challenges as well as learn the different ways of overcoming these challenges. Other people's success stories could sound like they are boasting about their achievements but to you, other people's success stories should be a blueprint to your own success.

With the presence of social media, people from across the world have found a platform on which to share their success with others who are starting or continuing on the Ketogenic diet. Instagram has numerous hashtags that people have created to share with others on their success after adopting the Ketogenic diet for various reasons. #ketotransformation and #ketofam are examples of hashtags on Instagram that have been started so that people from across the globe can share their stories to motivate others.

An Instagram page by the name *ketosuccessforbeginners* on 5th October 2019 published, on their page, a story of a woman who is on the Ketogenic diet and has already lost 100 pounds and still continuing the diet to achieve her goal of losing more weight. Her story is quoted below;

"What a year this has been. I can honestly say that this has been my best and happiest year in 8 years. From dealing with my dad's cancer and losing him, to a failed engagement, to college struggled due to my grief, gaining over 100 pounds, moving, and moving and moving again, major mental and physical health struggles and an uncertain future and a job that made me miserable to getting healthy and living my best life. I wish I had known the difference that would be made in all parts of my life just by putting my health first. I started with that and the rest just fell into place. I'll always be grateful to Keto for being the tool that allowed me to get to where I am now. It's scary to think where I would be had I not found it. I'm so grateful to all of you and I sincerely wish you the best year ever in 2019. Here's to the New Year! Tag me in your 2018 transformation pictures! I want to celebrate YOU. Sometimes some posts just bring out trolls. Don't interact with them! Remember that happy people will lift people up, not try to knock them down. If you've been following me you've seen my transformation in real-time via videos on my story. I'm still barely out of the 300 pounds if I were lying about anything, I would definitely try to lie about that. I still have a very long way to go. I post just as many bad things as good- the bloats the gains, the stalls. All of it. If people want to discredit the hard work because they're too sad to believe it's possible, let them. Love y'all!"

This story is meant to motivate you to surge on and shut your ears to the negatives that other people could be saying about you.

Another Instagram user, *kristina.nicole13* on 21st January 2018 published a story about how she used the Ketogenic diet to achieve her target weight. Her story is meant to inspire you to do the same and get started on that diet. Her story is quoted below;

"I used to be seriously overweight for a time of my life (likely viewed as corpulent). A few people have known me quite a while and have seen my progress, however, some have only known me now and don't have a clue of what I used to be. There are a couple of long periods of my being with zero to not many pictures of me since I loathed the manner in which I looked. After leaving a not so healthy relationship (when I ate my emotions out of sadness), I had the chance to lose a tad all alone by concentrating on #me and getting once again into activities I enjoyed (musical theater) and in general, being glad once more. However, I was as yet overweight and kind of hit a level, so I lost hope on the grounds that nothing appeared to work. It wasn't until October of 2016 that I found out about the #ketogenic way of life and began that method of eating and had the option to shed 10 pounds in 2 months, just from settling on better nourishment decisions. In January of 2017, I started a wellness system, setting off to the #gym around 4-6 days in a week of doing a blend of weight lifting and cardio. My hope was to hit my #goal weight in one year. Frankly, I didn't think I would do it, but I made a promise to myself that I would be glad in the event that I drew near.) It's been a year since I did my first #workout all alone and I am so excited to state that I did it. I hit my target weight! Since June of 2015 to date, I have shed around 76 pounds/7 dress sizes and I'm a more joyful, more advantageous, and more grounded rendition of myself than I have ever been in my life! It is not only about the number and my physical, but I have also discovered that I have to deal with my body mentally and physically for #health reasons as well. I currently have more vitality and I feel completely stunning. I at last feel like the rendition of myself that I constantly imagined in my mind. It has been a tedious and difficult road to where I am and there were several moments I wanted to give up. I'm posted my photos not out of pride, but since I'm simply so #happy that I did it and I need individuals to realize that they can do whatever they set their focus on!!"

Tippywyatt, another Instagram user, also on April 5th, 2018 published her experiences on the Ketogenic diet. Take a look at her experience below;

"This is my 31-Day Keto Diet Change! The past couple of months of 2017 were challenging for me. With such a large number of life changes occurring, I wound up at the edge of mental and physical weariness. Keeping so much to myself, I allowed my worries to get the better part of me. I began to disregard my wellbeing in manners I haven't done in years. I frantically required positive change. I urgently required my old self back. I talk about the appalling reactions that transpired during those 3 months of disregard and my 31-day Keto diet voyage to reset my way of life. You can watch my YouTube video or read my blog entry on my site (tippytales.com) for more information on the Keto diet, how I approached doing it, my fair assessment, my outcomes, my present status 2 months post my reset and on the off chance that I am making it a way of life. Putting yourself out there and posting before and after photos is startling for many individuals. I am indistinguishable to this idea yet I expected to share this. Why? Without a doubt since I am pleased and I realize how hard I attempted to get myself back. Despite the fact that how I feel changed, I realized the greater change is inside. I can wholeheartedly say I cherish my body and the lady I've moved towards becoming from this battle to get myself back. On the off chance that this motivates one individual to have confidence in themselves somewhat more today than yesterday then these arrangements of ungainly postures filled its need. We are generally human and now and again we have difficulties throughout everyday life. I accept mishaps are there which is as it should be. To test us. To test how gravely we genuinely and profoundly need it. Plus, what's a decent story without a stellar rebound?! Not a decent one as I would like to think."

This is another success story that was published by another Instagram user. Take a look at their success and feel motivated.

"2 years, 70 pounds less. I've changed more than just physically since this time but to be honest I'm really proud of myself. In 2016 I was 205 pounds and as of today, I've lost 70. I think my current weight (135) is pretty good for 5 '10." I've gone from size 15 jeans to size 2/4, I've worked so hard and now I can see it. 2 years later I'm so different in ways I never would have guessed. Thank you to everyone who supported me but more than that thanks to everyone who poked fun at me because without you guys, I would have never made this change for myself. It was lost healthily and one of the most difficult things. I'm still not 100% confident but I feel so much better and I'm fine with slightly bragging about this. No matter what others say, only you can define your worth. So, from a 1X to a small, from 2016 to 2018, and from my life then to my life now, if there's one thing I learned is that hard work will eventually pay off. "

And lastly, another success story of a woman who lost weight while on the Ketogenic diet and who is being celebrated by others.

KetoVale

Now I am super excited to share an amazing Keto success journey Elena Juarez aka @thestairlady. In a span of one year, Elena managed to lose 100 pounds on Keto. Not only did she achieve this incredible success with Keto, but the members of her family are experiencing great results.

Read her full story on our website KetoVale.com @KetoVale for motivation and tips! (Article link: https://www.ketovale.com/elena-juarezs-keto-success-story/) or simply Google "Elena Juarez KetoVale" for the article.

CHAPTER 4
CHEESE AND A HEALTHY KETOGENIC MEAL

Definition Of Cheese

You probably already know that cheese is a dairy product that is obtained from milk. It consists of casein, a milk protein, and can be produced in several distinct flavors. Cheese is made up of protein and fat and is usually from the milk produced by either sheep, goats, buffaloes, or cows. During the production process of cheese, the milk from these animals is acidified. Rennet, a type of enzyme, is added to the acidified milk leading to coagulation. Calcium, fat, protein, and phosphorus are nutrients present in cheese. Cheese is also known for its ability to last for long periods of time life compared to regular milk.

Types Of Cheese

There are numerous known brands of cheese across cultures in the world and because of this cheese is classified by; method of making and its length of life, texture, animal milk, place of origin, fat content.

Health Benefits Of Using Cheese

As stated earlier, cheese is rich in nutrients such as calcium, fat, and iron which for you on a Keto diet is essential. Similarly, cheese contains zinc, phosphorus, and vitamins some of the most essential requirement for the human body. Cheese, a dairy product, could be better positioned to protect your teeth from cavities.

According to research and study, some types of cheese comprise bits of conjugated linoleic acid which may help your body against obesity and heart diseases. The calcium in cheese is responsible for strengthening your bones. Cheese, through its containment of vitamin B, is essential in maintaining a healthy and glowing youthful skin.

Risks Associated With The Consumption Of Cheese

Cheese does not have fiber and the ingestion of large amounts could lead to constipation. If you are a lactose-intolerant person, the consumption of cheese could be a challenge for you. This is because cheese comprises of lactose which your body might not be able to digest since it lacks the accountable enzymes for breaking it down. Worry not! Some types of cheese, parmesan, are low in lactose which might be a benefit if you are a lactose intolerant individual. Casein is a milk protein that you may be sensitive to and even the low lactose cheese may not be suggested for you.

Recommended Cheese For A Healthy Keto Diet

Mozzarella cheese which contains;

- 5.5g of proteins
- 86 Calories
- 1g of carbs
- 142 mg of calcium
- 6g fat

Feta cheese which contains;

- 4g of fat
- 61 Calories
- 5g of protein
- 1g of carbs
- 59g Calcium

Herbs and Spices and a Healthy Ketogenic Meal

Definition of Herbs and Spices

In simple words, herbs are the leafy parts of a plant that are flavorsome when they remain and get used fresh. Herbs massively grow in mild regions all over the world. On the other hand, spices are the opposite of herbs. They are not leafy rather any other part of the plant. For instance, asafetida is a gum, cumin is a fruit and peppercorns are berries. Usually, spices are used in low quantities and are more nutritional when they are dried. The drying procedure takes place directly after harvesting the spices. They are dried in either drying rooms or right under the sun. Once dried, the spices are stored in sealed containers so as to reserve their oils that are responsible for the flavor in meals. One plant can be both a spice and an herb.

Brief History of Herbs and Spices

Herbs and spices have been used by human beings long before civilization and are still a vital part of the human diet to date. They were used as additives or simply to add flavor to the meals of the early man. Though with contemporary ways of preserving foods, the role of herbs and spices has been condensed to flavoring foods and for medicinal purposes. Early Egyptians mummified the bodies of their treasured ones with herbs and spices. Cardamom was used by the Romans and the Greeks to help in digestion during and after meals while the Indians used it as a curative herb to fight ailments. Garlic was administered by different cultures across the world to laborers as a way of boosting their strength. Across the world, herbs and spices have been used by man for numerous reasons because of their varying abilities. Today, you are certain to find herbs and spices all over shelves in stores or in open markets and are still used for the same purposes.

Why Herbs and Spices?

Modern science has proved that herbs and spices have health remunerations to you if you are using them. For example, cinnamon lowers the body's blood sugar level, peppermint is beneficial in relieving pain and also curbs nausea, basil improves your immune system putting you in a better place to fight illnesses and ginger is known for treating nausea. Alternatively, garlic improves the heart as well as combats sickness while cayenne pepper has anti-cancer properties that are essential for you in the avoidance and combating of cancer.

Side Effects of Herbs and Spices

It is easy to ignore that herbs and spices have side effects albeit all the advantages and benefits. Garlic has additive effects will ginger causes bleeding the iris. Other side effects include; nervousness, high blood pressure, violence and at times psychotic behavior, vomiting, delusions, confusion and suspicion, tremors, seizures, renal failure, rapid heart rates, unconsciousness and even at times demise.

Fruits And Vegetables And A Healthy Ketogenic Meal
What Are Fruits And Vegetables?

Essentially vegetables are plant parts that are eatable by man as food. The parts include stems, seeds or even flowers. Potatoes and carrots are classified as vegetables since they are edible by human beings. Vegetables are a central part of any meal since they offer vitamins D, B, C, A, carbohydrates and minerals which are vital for the body in general. Some of the common vegetables worldwide include; potatoes, broccoli, carrots, cabbage (red and green) spinach, legumes, lettuce, onions, and tomatoes.

Fruits are fleshy and frequently the sweet parts of a certain plant that has seeds in them and are edible by man. Human beings across time have depended on fruits as a source of food as well as a way of continuing the growth of plants by replanting the seeds found in the fruits. Most fruits are edible by man in their raw state and may not require any form of cooking before ingesting. Some of the common fruits across cultures in the world include; bananas, oranges, grapes, strawberries, and apples

Botanically speaking, cereal grains are at times considered as fruits, but their fruit walls are so thin that they are attached to the cereal's seed coat making them seeds. For instance; corn and wheat

Fruits And Vegetables That Support The Ketogenic Diet

However, most fruits are high in carbs and therefore they are often ignored during a Keto diet plan. However, berries are low in carbs and wealthier in fiber making them friendly to the Keto diet. Berries (raspberries, strawberries, blackberries, and blueberries) carry antioxidants that are important in the human body in that they protect you against diseases.

Vegetables are very healthy and are very good for you. If and only if you are on the Keto diet should you worry about vegetables. As stated in this cookbook the Keto diet backs a high in fat and low in carbs diet plan, you might want to do away with some vegetables that are high in carbs. Carrots and potatoes (sweet potatoes as well as regular potatoes) are high in starch and could possibly interfere with the ketosis process even when ingested in small quantities. Instead, spinach, bell peppers, zucchini, cauliflower, cabbage, broccoli, asparagus, celery, arugula, onion, olives, and pumpkins are all Keto-friendly and thus, recommended for your usage.

What To Avoid

As much as fruits and vegetables offer health benefits to the human body, the fact that they are rich in carbs puts them off when you are on the Keto diet. Apples, watermelons, mangoes, limes, cherries, pineapples, bananas, oranges, grapes, and plums are some of the fruits that could interfere with your ketogenic meal plan. Beets, potatoes (both sweet and regular) yams, turnips are some of the vegetables whether ingested in small quantities could disrupt the Keto diet plan. You should be in a position to know the kind of fruits that are Keto friendly in order to maintain your ketosis.

Why The Ketogenic Fruit And Vegetable Bread?

Any diet rich in fruits and vegetables, the Ketogenic fruit and vegetable bread included, is beneficial to you in that it lowers your chances of suffering from heart diseases. The dietary fiber contained in vegetables is important because it is responsible for the lowering of your body's blood cholesterol levels and reduce your risk of heart diseases. This bread offers you a chance to reduce your chances of developing cardiovascular diseases

This bread also gives you a chance to minimize your chances of coming into contact with cancer. You already know that cancer is deadly and the mere fact that the bread offers you a shield against cancer should be reason enough for you to bake and consume. The Keto fruit and vegetable bread also lowers your chances of developing prostate cancer if you are a man.

The Keto fruit and vegetable bread also lowers your risk of contracting diabetes.

The fiber in these fruits and vegetable bread is essential in ensuring your digestive system is smooth.

Gluten And A Healthy Ketogenic Meal
What Is A Gluten-Free Meal?

Gluten is a result of protein called prolamin and glutelins found in most cereal grains. This protein is what adds up to 75-85% of all the protein found in wheat as well as other cereals related to wheat such as oats, barley and also found in products made from these cereals such as malts and bread. A gluten-free meal in simple terms is a meal that has successfully excluded gluten.

A gluten-free diet should be one that is naturally

gluten-free. Egg, milk, nuts, fruits, vegetables, potatoes, rice, and dairy products that have a better balance of macro and micronutrients are relevant and essential for a glutton free diet.

You may wonder why a gluten-free meal is essential. The gluten-free meal is essential in that the meal is a treatment for celiac disease and other medical conditions that are a result of gluten.

It is also a very important thing to always check for labels when buying foods from supermarkets if you are allergic to gluten. The label "gluten-free" would do be on most products with no gluten. You should also ask if the foods you are buying have come into any form of contact with other food that contain gluten in order to avoid an allergic reaction later on.

Why The Ketogenic Gluten-Free Bread?

As stated earlier, a naturally gluten-free meal is essential in that gluten proteins to have minimal nutritional value and thus, it is actually healthier to ingest the gluten-free bread. This is because it improves the cholesterol levels reducing your chances of heart-related diseases, certain cancer, and diabetes. The gluten-free bread promotes healthy weight loss as well as improving your health if you have arthritis and helps you to ward off germs because the bread offers antioxidants, minerals, and vitamins. This bread is good news for you if you have a gluten allergy because you no longer have to worry about the problem.

The gluten-free bread also enhances digestion as well as improves your energy levels. This bread is also beneficial to you in that it eliminates processed foods from your diet; for instance, fried foods that are actually unhealthy for you. This bread offers you a chance to eat healthy and will ensure that your body remains healthy as well.

What To Eat That Is Gluten-Free

- Tapioca
- Most dairy products (cream, cheese, yogurt, milk)
- Fresh eggs
- Fruits and vegetables
- Nuts and seeds
- Fish
- Poultry
- Unprocessed beans

What To Avoid

- Beer
- Regular bread
- Soups
- Fries (French fries)
- Cereals such as malt, barley, and wheat)
- Candies
- Processed meat
- Milkshakes
- Pasta
- Pies and cakes

Cons Of A Gluten-Free Diet

You might experience digestive issues as a result of insufficient consumption of fiber. Constipation could be a major challenge for you in that a gluten-free meal has little to no fiber.

You could also experience rapid weight gain as a result of ingesting gluten-free products that are usually high in fats and sugar. Furthermore, you could as well experience weight gain as your intestinal track attempts to recover and properly start to absorb nutrients.

Despite the fact that celiac disease is treated by adopting and sticking to the gluten-free meal, it could be a problem for you to find gluten-free meals especially if you are opting to eat out.

Any damage in your intestines could take longer periods of time to heal or fail to heal it all. Failing in the maintenance of a gluten-free meal could possibly mean you will suffer from osteoporosis (a disease that is associated with the bones) or even cancer at large. It may also have occurred to you that a regular gluten-free meal is more expensive than a regular meal.

Sweeteners And A Healthy Ketogenic Diet What are Sweeteners?

A sweetener is any substance that has the same function as sugar in either foods or drinks but is used to sweeten the drinks and foods in the place of regular sugar. For example, there artificial and natural sweeteners.

Types Of Sweeteners That Support The Keto Diet

As stated earlier in this cookbook, ketogenic diets

advocate for cutting back in high carbs foods for example processed snacks. This is important for you if you want your body to reach the ketosis stage and burn fat instead of carbs to produce energy for your body. Ketosis is also a result of low sugar consumption which could pose a challenge if you want to sweeten your bread. Lucky for you there are actually low carb sweeteners that support the Keto diet.

- ***Xylitol*** - This is a type of sugar alcohol that is usually found in candies, sugar-free gum as well as mints. You may use this sweetener to bake, but you would need more liquids because it tends to increase dryness in the dough as a result of its moisture-absorbent nature. The carbs in this sweetener do not raise your blood sugar levels or insulin levels, unlike the regular sugar, does.

  Note: *Xylitol, when used in high amounts, may cause digestive issues; thus, you should be careful with the amounts you use.*

- ***Sucralose*** - this sweetener passes through your body undigested simply because it is a non-metabolized artificial sweetener that it has no carbs or calories making it popular on the markets since it lacks the bitter test common in many artificial sweeteners.

Note: *When exposed to high temperatures this sweetener is known to produce compounds that may be harmful to your body; therefore, it is not recommended for baking purposes. Instead, you could use sucralose as a low carb way of sweetening your foods and drinks.*

- ***Stevia*** – This is a natural sweetener that contains very little amount of carbs or calories. It is from the <u>stevia rebaudiana</u> plant and unlike the regular sugar stevia may be useful in lowering blood sugar levels. This sweetener can be found in both the liquids and the powder states and you could use it to sweeten your food or drinks.

Note: *Stevia is much sweeter than regular sugar; thus, you should be careful with the amounts you desire in either your food or drinks or even when using it in a recipe.*

- ***Monk fruit sweetener*** – It is a natural sweetener and it contains no calories as well as no carbs which is an essential element in the maintenance of a ketogenic diet. This sweetener is extracted from a plant in China called the monk fruit. The sweetness of this natural sweetener is a result of the natural compounds and sugars, which are antioxidants. This sweetener is essential for regulating blood sugar levels in your body.

Note: *You could decide to use the monk fruit sweetener in the place of regular sugar, but you should be in a position to reduce the amount of the sweetener in half in order to achieve the required results.*

What Sweeteners To Avoid While On A Low-Carb Carb Diet

These sweeteners may interfere with the ketosis process because they are high in carbs and could increase the sugar levels in your blood.

- *Maple syrup* – this is a good sweetener because it carries with it good amounts of zinc and manganese, essential for the body, but it is high in sugar as well as high in carbs.

- *Honey* – this is a natural sweetener that has a lot of benefits on the human body making it more recommended than the regular sugar, but it is high in calories and carbs making it a poor decision when on the Keto diet.

- ***Dates*** – this is a natural sweetener that has amounts of fiber, minerals, and vitamins, essential in the human body, but they are high in carbs.

- ***Coconut sugar*** – this sweetener is a result of the coconut palm and is usually absorbed more slowly compared to the regular sugar, but it is still high in fructose which is bad for the regulation of blood sugar levels in the body.

- ***Agave nectar*** - This sweetener, when consumed, reduces your body's sensitivity to insulin and makes it harder for your body to regulate its blood sugar levels.

- ***Maltodextrin*** – This sweetener is a highly processed one which is high in calories and carbs just like the regular sugar. It is made from plants with lots of starch, for instance, corn and rice.

Why Sweeteners Instead Of Regular Sugar?

You might probably be asking yourself this very question. Well, the answer is simple. Sweeteners, like the regular sugar, provide a sweet test during consumption, but what sweeteners have over regular sugar is the ability to not increase the body's blood sugar levels. Extensive conduction of research studies has proven that sweeteners are safe for consumption on a daily basis. For instance, if you are suffering from diabetes the use of sweetness is useful to you because you do not have to worry about your body's blood sugar levels when you are out enjoying your meals with family and friends.

Nutritional Facts On A Healthy Keto Meal

Carbohydrates take the greatest percentage of regular meals across the world. However, the Ketogenic diet discourages the consumption of foods rich in carbohydrates but instead, it advocates for foods rich in fats and moderate in protein. We are going to look at the nutritional facts of what is termed as a healthy Ketogenic diet.

On a normal diet, human beings consume up to 50% to 55% of carbohydrates. That is more than half the percentage of the whole meal. Proteins take up about 25% of the remaining meal while fats take up the remaining 20%. This is contrary to the Ketogenic diet which constitutes about 75% of fats, 20% of protein and only 5% of carbohydrates. For instance, if you weigh 160 pounds and you are averagely active, then your body would require approximately 30 grams of carbohydrates, 90 grams of protein and 200 grams of fats for a single day while on the Ketogenic diet.

- **Cholesterol;** is an organic molecule and is important in the structure of the cell membranes. The normal cholesterol levels in an adult are less than *200 mg/dl (milligrams per deciliter)*. The Ketogenic diet has been reported to regulate the cholesterol levels of some people who adopted the diet. The diet decreases the levels of triglycerides, blood sugar as well as LDL cholesterol.

- **Protein;** it is recommended to ingest between 0.6 – 1.0 grams of protein per pound in the weight of your body (1.6 – 2.0 grams per kilogram). Note that consuming protein in large amounts could get your body out of ketosis.

- **Fat;** the levels of calories originating from fats will depend on how low your consumption of carbohydrates is and this is probably between 55 – 80%. You could consume;

- *1,600 calories for about 85 – 130*

grams of fat in a day.

- *2,000 calories for about 115 – 170 grams of fat in a day.*
- *2,500 calories for about 140 – 210 grams of fat in a day.*

- **Carbohydrates;** it should be noted that there is no set limit for carbs in a Ketogenic diet. However, anything below 100 grams is considered low carb. You could achieve ketosis is you ate unprocessed real foods.

- **Sugar;** Ketogenic diet ensures you abstain from all foods with carbs including refined sugar. This means sugar should be limited as low as possible to ensure your body gets into nutritional ketosis.

- **Grain and dairy;** grains and dairy products are rich in carbs which is against the Ketogenic diet meaning you have to minimize your consumption to fit in the daily less than 100 grams of carbs.

- **Vitamins;** vegetables such as kale, spinach and broccoli are Keto friendly. They are rich in vitamin A. 1 ounce of beef liver should provide up to 5% of vitamin A. vitamin B is provided by red meat or nuts and seed and could be a good addition to the diet. Vitamin C is also found in broccoli and spinach which should have you covered in that front. Vitamin E is provided by nuts and seeds while vitamin K is catered for by olive oil and beef.

- **Minerals;** *calcium* should be supplemented in the body when your body is attempting to adapt to the diet as the diet could flash out the nutrients when your body is still adapting to the diet. *Chloride* is another mineral that should be ingested in elevated levels when your body is still adapting to the Keto diet. It is found in abundance in table salt or even sea salt. *Chromium* is possibly a mineral that could lack in your Keto diet. This is because most foods only have 12mcg per serving and are found in broccoli. Chromium is easily excreted when your body is still adapting to the diet. *Copper* is another mineral that is abundant in the Ketogenic diet. It is mainly found in seeds, nuts, chocolate (dark) or even seafood. *Fluoride* is another mineral that is found mostly in water as well as greens and avocados. *Iodine* is another mineral that is found in the Ketogenic diet abundant in seafood specifically the white fish or eggs as well as dairy. *Iron* is another mineral that should be ingested and is found in animal products for instance meat. **Magnesium** is also found in seafood and meat. Magnesium intake should be increased as your body still attempts to adapt to the Ketogenic diet. You could also use magnesium supplements to supplement the nutrient in the body. Magnesium speeds up your body into getting into ketosis and assists your body to transition from the normal diet to the Ketogenic diet. **Manganese** is present in large quantities in spices and also in seafood, nuts, or seeds. **Phosphorus** can be found in nuts, meats or even dairy and is not lacking in the Ketogenic diet. **Potassium** is greatly found in meats, in Keto-friendly vegetables, seafood as well as in avocados. Just like most nutrients, potassium intake needs to be increased because the diet could excrete a lot of it when your body is still adapting to the Ketogenic diet. **Selenium** is found in abundance in Brazil nuts as well as in yellowfin tuna as well as animal products. **Sodium** is another major mineral that is found in salt and is very much present in your Ketogenic diet. Just like most minerals, you need to increase your consumption as Sodium could largely be excreted when your body is adapting to the diet. You could opt to sprinkle table salt over your food as a way of supplementing the mineral. **Sulfur** is found in eggs and a lot of Keto friendly vegetables have it. **Zinc** is contained in seafood as well as meat and you could also find it in nuts and dairy.

- **Other nutrients;** *fiber* is another important nutrient that you should ingest when you are on the Ketogenic diet to prevent constipation. Plant products are the best source of fiber, for instance, avocados, nuts as well as seeds.

CHAPTER 5
REGULARLY ASKED QUESTIONS ABOUT THE KETOGENIC DIET

It should be noted that having doubts about the effectiveness of the diet or asking numerous questions about it is completely normal. This book will attempt to answer several regularly asked questions for you. However, it is recommended that you should visit your doctor or nutritionist for more information concerning the Ketogenic diet. Your doctor will be in a better position to answer your questions and provide you with information that could be left out in this book.

Why Is It Important To Stick To The Ketogenic Meal Plan?

We have tackled this topic several times in this book already. However, the question 'why is it important to stick to the Ketogenic diet 'keeps coming up all the time. As we stated earlier, the Ketogenic diet has numerous benefits to you once you have decided to start on it. Let us find an answer to this recurring question.

The Ketogenic diet is important because;

- **It reduces your blood's insulin and sugar levels;** if you are suffering from diabetes, the Ketogenic diet is very helpful. Doing away with carbohydrates is proven to reduce your blood sugar levels drastically. This also reduces your insulin levels in the blood. This is however efficient if you have visited and consulted with your doctor and they have suggested the Ketogenic meal plan for you. This diet could even remedy type 2 diabetes.

- **It lowers your body's blood pressure;** hypertension is a great risk factor to you in that you could contact other diseases such as stroke, kidney failure or even heart-related diseases. However, sticking to the Ketogenic diet could prove beneficial in that doing away with carbohydrates lowers your blood pressure and thus, reduces your chances of contracting the mentioned diseases and could possibly assist you to live longer.

- **It improves your LDL Cholesterol levels**; if you have high LDL cholesterol levels, you stand a great risk of contracting heart-related diseases including possible heart attacks. This depends on the particle size of the LD. If you have large particles, then your chances of suffering from a heart attack are low whilst having small particles increases your risk of suffering from a possible heart attack. The Ketogenic diet increases the LDL particles in size in your blood. Thus, if you opt to lower your consumption of carbohydrates, you are improving your chances of avoiding a possible heart attack.

- **It is a therapy for brain disorders;** glucose is very important for your brain in its day to day functioning. Your brain burns glucose to provide energy for it to function normally. Once you adopt the Ketogenic diet, your body's liver is forced to produce glucose from the protein you ingest. However, your brain can also burn ketones, which are a result of the Ketogenic diet. This way, the diet remedies epilepsy in children who are unresponsive to the drugs related to epilepsy. The diet could be a possible cure for epilepsy. The diet is also known for its ability to remedy Alzheimer's disease as well as Parkinson's disease.

- **It lowers your body's triglycerides;** if you are wondering what triglycerides are, they are fat molecules that move in your blood. It has been proven that high levels of triglycerides could lead to heart-related diseases. These levels are elevated in your body if you consume high amounts of carbohydrates and thus, the diet comes in handy and assists you in cutting your carbs consumption. Additionally, consuming low fats could also raise the levels of triglycerides in your blood which means the Ketogenic diet appropriate to stick to.

- **It assists you in shedding weight;** as we stated earlier in this book, this diet is an effective agent in your attempts to lose weight. Cutting carbohydrates in your diet in the most effective way for you to lose weight. Low carb diets are very effective in weight loss because of their ability to get rid of excess water in your body in the process lowering your body's insulin levels, which in turn speeds up your weight loss. This is however effective in the short-term weight loss and not so effective for the long-term plan. This is why it is important to seek your physician's opinion before embarking on the diet.

- **It reduces your appetite;** the Ketogenic diet is important in reducing your appetite if you are trying to fight obese. Hunger is what leads to overeating and becoming obese in the end. Cutting carbohydrates in your meal and ingesting more fats and proteins leads to consuming fewer calories. Doing away with carbohydrates is one way to minimize your appetite as well as your intake of calories.

In conclusion, if you are looking to boost your blood's sugar and insulin levels or if you are looking to lose appetite, lose weight, lower your triglycerides, remedying brain disorders, lowering your blood pressure or becoming healthier in general, you have all the reasons to stick to the diet.

How Long Would It Take For The Ketogenic Diet To Be Effective?

By now you already know that the Ketogenic diet is among the world's famous low carbohydrates diet. The diet is responsible for the reason why your body no longer burns carbohydrates instead it burns fats to produce ketones that are responsible for the day to day functioning of your body. After adopting the diet, the question 'how long until you enter ketosis 'begs for attention. Most people get worried that they might not enter ketosis in time and thus, they tend to give up on the diet as a result.

The fact is that the amount of time it would take you to enter ketosis is not the same amount of time someone else could need to get into ketosis. Additionally, many people find it hard for their bodies to enter ketosis. Let us take a look at how long it could possibly take you to enter ketosis.

In order for you to benefit from the diet, your body needs to get into ketosis first. Ketosis, as we defined it earlier, is a state that your body adapts to when it starts burning fats into molecules which we referred to as ketones. Ketones are your body's main source of energy once your body stops burning carbohydrates to produce glucose, usually the main source of energy on the normal diet.

The first step that you would take as a way of reaching ketosis is doing away with carbohydrates. It is important to note that your body stores excess glucose in your liver or your muscles. The glucose is stored in its storage form, glycogen. Switching to burning fats by your body could take time because your body would be required to burn all the glucose in your body before opting to burn fats for energy. The time required for your body to successfully make this change is different from everyone else. This could be because of varying carbohydrates intake in your daily meals as well as varying consumptions of proteins, fats or how regularly you exercise your body, your age or even your body's metabolism rates.

For instance, if you consume carbohydrates in large or elevated levels, once you have started on the Ketogenic diet, your body could take longer before it gets into ketosis. This is contrary to your consumption of carbohydrates as an average or lower consumer. It would take you a shorter time compared to the high levels of carbohydrates consumers to get into ketosis. This is because your body would be required to finish all its glucose in the body including the stored glycogen. The more carbohydrates you consume, the more the stored glycogen and the more the amount of time required to completely burn it in your body.

It would require you between 2 to 5 days, if you are an average consumer of carbohydrates, to get into ketosis. This is approximate if you consume 50 to 60 grams of carbohydrates in a day. The duration of time could be altered depending on a number of factors including; the body's metabolism, your age, your level of physical activity as well as your protein, carbohydrates, and fat intake.

You will be able to tell if you are on ketosis if you experienced a number of symptoms including the Ketogenic flu. You could experience nausea, bad breath, elevated thirst, or fatigue. These are possible ways to tell if you are already in ketosis. However, the most accurate and reliable source of knowledge on your ketosis level is if you test your body of the ketone levels. You could opt to visit your doctor or physician and they would run a few tests on you to determine the ketone levels in your body. Or you could measure the Beta-hydroxybutyrate levels using the ketone meter at the comfort of your house.

Some people take longer to get into ketosis because they most probably ingest carbohydrates without knowing. Consuming carbohydrates could possibly hinder the rate at which it would require your body to get into ketosis. It could as well get your body out of ketosis in the process. There is no standard limit to limit your consumption of carbohydrates to ensure that your body gets into ketosis. Different people could get into ketosis by eating different levels of carbohydrates, you included. This is why it is important to consult with your doctor. Another possible reason could be that you are not ingesting the required levels of fats in your diet. The Ketogenic advocates for up to 70% of fats to be consumed as well as 20% of protein and possibly 5% or 10% of carbohydrates. Changing or altering this ratio could possibly mean you will take longer to get into ketosis. Other reasons could be your age, physical exercise levels, personal stress or even lack of adequate sleep. These could possibly affect the rate at which your body could get into ketosis.

You could improve your chance of getting into ketosis if you exercised regularly, minimize your carbohydrates consumption, increasing your fat consumption or even by testing your ketone levels regularly.

Is It Possible To Gain Weight While On The Ketogenic Diet?

Despite the fact that the Ketogenic diet is responsible for a healthy way of losing weight, the diet could be responsible for your gaining of weight. By talking about the Ketogenic diet, we are actually talking about the increased consumption of fats. You could possibly gain weight on the diet without your knowledge.

We are going to analyze and examine the possible ways the diet could lead your body into gaining more weight.

You may not be taking care of your body; it does not matter what diet you are on if you are not indulging your body in any physical activities or sleeping enough, chances are high that you will gain weight. Stress is another factor that could lead to weight gain while on the Ketogenic diet. It is recommended to stay away from stress while on the Ketogenic diet. Stress may lead to your body secreting cortisol which is the reason why you gain weight instead of losing it.

You are not properly following the diet and its rules; if for instance you are sliding and falling into eating foods that are high in carbohydrates knowingly or unknowingly could lead to weight gain instead of weight loss while on the diet. Sabotaging the diet by any means could lead to a possible weight gain if you do not notice or realize it.

You are encouraging 'cheat days 'on your diet; 'cheat days 'are the days you convince yourself that avoiding the Ketogenic diet could not be harmful. You could probably consume high carb foods on these days and alter your body's ketosis. It is important to note that the Ketogenic diet does not make room for 'cheat days ' and thus, the risk of gaining weight while on the diet is increased. It is even worse if you are having many 'cheat days 'on your Ketogenic meal plan. This gets your body out of ketosis and the weight that you lost while you were faithful to the diet come back rushing and lead to weight gain.

You are including too many calories in your diet; it is actually very easy to consume a lot of calories while on the Ketogenic diet. It is very easy to lose track of your intake of calories when you are on the Ketogenic diet. This could, in turn, lead to weight gain instead of weight loss. To avoid this risk, it is important to keep track of your calories. You could visit your doctor and have them determine the levels of calories in your body.

You are not eating enough; regulating your consumption of calories does not necessarily mean that you should stop on calories completely. Your body could get out of ketosis if there are no adequate calories in your diet and this could lead to weight gain instead of weight loss. Inadequate consumption of calories could greatly stall your weight loss process if you are on the Ketogenic diet.

You are consuming alcohol; it is important to note that alcohol has carbs that could possibly hinder your Ketogenic diet. Most beers have elevated levels of sugars which is high in carbs and could lead to weight gain instead of weight loss if you are on the diet.

You are consuming too much fat; being on the Ketogenic diet does not necessarily mean that you get to consume a lot of fats. This could lead to weight gain in the end. Too much consumption of foods can lead to weight gain, fats included. Fats are rich in calories and altering the ratio that your body requires could lead to weight gain. It is recommended to consume fats that are stipulated on your diet and stick to that. Altering the ratio and adding too much fat, dense in calories could lead to weight gain.

You are consuming too much protein; consuming too much protein could possibly get your body out of ketosis. This is a process referred to as gluconeogenesis which entails the transformation of excess proteins into glycogen and is stored in your body which reverses your body's dependency on ketones to glucose. This could lead to unwanted weight gain in the end. It is advisable to consume the amount of proteins stipulated in your diet.

You are ignoring most sources of carbohydrates; it is important to note that most foods have carbohydrates and ignoring this fact could possibly lead to weight gain. Most vegetables are rich in carbohydrates as well as fruits. Including vegetables and fruits that are not Keto-friendly could lead to weight gain. It is important to be in a position to know all foods that have carbohydrates and eat healthy while in on the Ketogenic diet.

The Ketogenic diet is not working for you; it is possible that you are gaining weight on the diet because the die is not working for you. Just because the diet works effectively on someone else does not mean that it would work for you. It guarantees nothing to be precise. If the diet is not right for your body, then it is not going to be effective and the continued consumption of these fats if the diet is not appropriate for your body could lead to weight gain. It is important to visit and consult with your doctor before taking the diet head-on to determine if your genetics are in line with the diet.

What Is The Dirty Ketogenic Diet?

The regular Ketogenic diet as it has been stated numerous times in this book is that it advocates for about 70% of fats, 20% of protein and finally 10% of carbohydrates. The 'dirty Ketogenic diet 'follows these same rules. The only difference is that it does not focus its attention on where these fats, proteins or carbohydrates come from. This could mean instead of eating foods rich in good fast, you could opt to eat a bunless double cheeseburger. Unlike the Ketogenic diet which follows and advocates for healthy oils like coconut oil, the dirty Ketogenic diet allows you to consume pork rinds.

It is essential to note that the dirty Ketogenic diet is so tempting and could be so appealing at first glance. It is easy to feel tempted to let go of the healthy Ketogenic diet and opt to use the dirty Ketogenic diet basing your argument that it follows the same path as the Ketogenic diet. This could actually work and your body could possibly get into ketosis. However, you will lack some macronutrients in the dirty Ketogenic diet compared to the wide range of nutrients present in the Ketogenic diet. It is possible to miss out on minerals, vitamins or even enzymes if you drop the Ketogenic diet for the dirty Ketogenic diet. You already know that the macronutrients are responsible for keeping your body's immune system strong as well as help your body to function normally.

Doing away with these nutrients after adopting the dirty Ketogenic diet could leave your body vulnerable to diseases.

You are wondering if it is possible to lose weight while on the dirty Ketogenic diet. It is more likely that you will experience bloating, elevated cravings, inflammation and even weight gain if you get off of the Ketogenic diet. The dirty Ketogenic diet focuses its attention on processed foods that contain too much sodium which could, in turn, be upsetting for your health. It is possible for your body to get in ketosis while you are on the dirty Ketogenic diet, but there is a huge difference between you and one is on the Ketogenic diet.

It could be that the reason that you are opting for the dirty Ketogenic diet is that you cannot find time to prepare yourself a meal and so you opt to eat out. This book already covered a wide variety of healthy foods that you could eat out and maintain a healthy Ketogenic diet. You could opt to hire a private chef who would prepare you healthy Ketogenic meals instead of eating out and finding yourself adopting the dirty Ketogenic diet.

The dirty Ketogenic diet could sound like the real deal, but nothing beats the standard Ketogenic diet on so many fronts.

How Can I Tell If My Body Is In Ketosis?

There are numerous signs that would indicate that your body is in Ketosis. For instance, if you happen to wake up with a fruity metallic taste in your mouth after adopting the diet, it is evidence to indicate that your body is already manufacturing ketones and that you are already in ketosis. It is also possible to experience a mental sharpness if your body manufactures elevated levels of ketones.

However, the only way to be certain that your body is in ketosis is to medically test for the levels of ketones in your body. You could opt to visit your local physician or your local doctor who will then run a few tests on you to determine if your body is in ketosis. On the other hand, you could opt to self-test and test your urine using the urine test, your blood using the blood test or your breathe using the Breathalyzer and determine your body's levels of ketones.

What Could Possibly Put Me Out Of Ketosis And How Can I Quickly Get Myself Back Into Ketosis?

Getting your body out of ketosis is very easy. This is because your body could get out of ketosis immediately after a meal even if that meal contains small traces of carbohydrates and your body could revert to burning carbohydrates for energy for a few hours. This is why it is advisable to stick to the Ketogenic diet with discipline. However, this is all normal and you do not have to press the panic button already. This is because your body is designed to burn carbohydrates for energy and it will automatically revert to burning carbohydrates if some is available in your meal.

It is important to note that ingesting artificial ketones has not been fully clinically tested thus it is not recommended as way of getting your body back into ketosis. There are a few things that you could do to assist your body to get back into Ketosis and these include; integrating periods of fasting or consuming certain types of fats that are Keto friendly, like MCTs.

I Am A Physically Active Person, Can I Still Practice The Ketogenic Diet?

It is very easy to assume that your lack of ingesting carbohydrates could interfere with your body's production of energy which could in return affect your performance given that you are an active person. This assumption is not true. This is because, research conducted on the Ketogenic diet has proven that the ketones produced by your body can actually boost your performance.

However, if you are indulge your body in high intensity sporting activities, like playing basketball or playing soccer, it is important to note that your performance could reduce significantly. The diet is mostly effective to sporting activities such long distance marathons or endurance races. You should make an attempt to reduce your workout intensity or rather you should stay away from activities that demand a lot of glucose while your body is in transition to the Ketogenic diet.

What Is Ketogenic Adaptation And What Does It Feel Like?

The term 'Ketogenic Adaptation' simply refers to the transition of your body from primarily burning carbohydrates to produce glucose, to burning fats to produce ketone bodies to be used instead of glucose. It could take your body a few days, after adapting to the Ketogenic diet, to completely burn all the glucose in your body before shifting its attention to burning fats to produce ketone bodies.

During the Ketogenic Adaptation period, it is a possibility that you will experience symptoms of carbohydrates withdrawal at the beginning but once your body has adjusted to using fats to produce ketone bodies for energy, you will find your cravings for carbohydrates reducing.

Is Alcohol Appropriate While On The Ketogenic Diet?

Alcohol is rich in carbs. The Ketogenic diet advocates for a meal that is high in fats, moderate in protein and very low in carbohydrates. Alcohol is clearly defying that order and ratio.

Putting the topic about alcohol and the Ketogenic diet

aside for a minute, alcohol is not good for your health in so many ways. Consuming too much alcohol could lead to inflammatory damages. The liver could be greatly affected in its day to day activity of removing harmful and toxic substances from your body, alcohol included. Years and years of consumption of alcohol could possibly interfere with the liver and lead to its failure. This would mean that your body would no longer be able to excrete these toxic substances out of your body which could be very harmful to you in the end. The pancreas is another organ in your body that is greatly affected by the consumption of alcohol. The pancreas is responsible for regulating your body's insulin as well as glucose. Alcohol would possibly interfere with all this and a failed pancreas would mean raised sugar levels as well as an inability to produce insulin to use the sugar in your body. This could lead to you suffering from diabetes. Alcohol can also alter your body's nervous system. Consumption of alcohol for a longer period of time could lead to the altering of the coordination between your brain and your body. You could experience problems with your speech as well as your balance. Long term memories could be a problem for you to hang on. Alcohol, generally, is not good for your health.

With this knowledge, alcohol is not so good when you are observing the Ketogenic diet. This is because, despite the fact that alcohol will speed up your transition from the normal diet to ketosis, your liver will, in the end, start burning the alcohol for energy and get you out of ketosis. This could lead to a sowed weight loss.

For you to be able to maintain a Ketogenic diet that is healthy, you would have to be of sound mind. A healthy Ketogenic diet will require your full attention and focus. It is easy to order for pizza and get out of ketosis when you are drunk than when you are sound of mind. Your choice of liquor does not matter, what counts is that you are not of sound mind and you re vulnerable to making poor choices that could possibly affect your diet.

However, if you find yourself in a position where doing away with alcohol is a problem, there are options that you could choose from and still maintain your ketosis. Numerous **hard liquors** are about 40% in alcohol including whiskey, vodka, brandy, tequila, rum, and scotch as well as gin. These drinks comprise of little or no sugars of their own. This makes them Keto friendly. The challenge arises when you want to blend your drink with something besides alcohol to create a more pleasant drink. While the addition of water is Keto friendly, adding tonic water or soda to your liquor means an addition of carbs to your body. This will definitely get you out of ketosis. Fruit juice should also not be added to alcohol for the same reason that they are high in carbohydrates.

It could be that you are not a hard liquor lover, but

instead, a wine lover. There are **wines** that are Keto friendly for both red and white wines. For instance, dry wine is low in sugar and that makes it Keto friendly. Here are a few options you could choose from;

Keto-friendly dry white wines may include;

- Italian pinot grigio which has about 0.7 grams of carbs per one ounce.

- Sauvignon Blanc which has about 0.5 grams of carbs per one ounce.

- Pinot Blanc which has about 0.60 grams of carbs per one ounce.

Keto-friendly dry red wines may include;

- Merlot which has about 0.70 grams of carbs per one ounce.

- Pinot noir which has about 0.69 grams of carbs per one ounce.

- Cabernet sauvignon which has about 0.75 grams of carbs per one ounce.

Probably you are not a lover of both hard liquor as well as wines, but you are a big fan of beer. Well, beer is made up of barley, yeast, water, and hops meaning that beer is not Keto friendly. From its content, beer should be avoided at all costs. This is because, beer is made from the breaking down of barley into sugary maltose, this is what yeast acts on and ends up creating an elevated amount of sugar compared to wines and hard liquor. However, there is one beer you could opt to use which is gluten-free and low in carbs, the *Omission Ultimate Light Golden Ale.*

What Chinese Food You Could Eat When On The Ketogenic Diet?

If you are a lover of Chinese food and you are on the Ketogenic diet, this book has you covered. The first step to ensure that you have a great Keto friendly Chinese food is that you should plan your visit to a Chinese restaurant. It is important to decide how much carbohydrates you are planning on consuming. In this case, you are on the Ketogenic diet which means you will have to keep your carbohydrates consumption in line with the requirements of the diet. If the restaurant has provided its recipe online, you could opt to check it and be sure that the restaurant is offering a Keto friendly diet. You could also call and ask or you could even message the restaurant.

Here are a few options you could consider;

- Meat and vegetables combined with savory sauce could be a good option. They could have little or no carbs as well as added sugars in them making them Keto friendly. For example, chicken served with mushrooms, curry chicken as well as Szechuan pawns.

- Walnut chicken is another great option because it is not made with sugar or starch making it Keto friendly.

- The Mu Shu is another option that is Keto friendly in Chinese restaurants. You could enjoy the Mu Shu without wrappers because it is low on carbs.

- Steamed foods are also Keto friendly. These may include steamed fish served with Keto-friendly vegetables in the place of deep-fried foods.

- Opting to serve thin soups in the place of thick soups is a good option when you are on the Ketogenic diet. For example, you could order for the egg drop thin soup.

- You could order for the black bean sauce which is low on carbs and Keto friendly.

You could as well use your sense of taste to determine the sugar level in the restaurant and choose to eat healthy.

What to avoid in a Chinese restaurant;

Dishes

- Rice which is either steamed or fried. Rice is rich in carbs and thus, it is not Keto friendly and could get your body of ketosis.

- Egg rolls should definitely be avoided.

- Avoid ordering noodles. These may include; chow Mein noodles, chow fun noodles as well as lo Mein noodles.

- All types of breaded meats.

Sauces

- Oyster sauce.

- Both the sweet and sour sauces.

- Duck sauce.

- Plum sauce.

- Hoisin sauce

Additional Thoughts On The Ketogenic Diet For Women

By now, you should be in a position to make a decision on whether you want to start on the diet, if you are considering it, or keep going if you already started on it. The book has clearly and in detail explained almost all the pros and cons of the diet. The book has explained the benefits that come with adapting to the diet as well as the types of meals you could consider eating and those you could possibly avoid. The book has also explained how you get into a healthy ketosis and benefit from the diet.

At this juncture, it is upon you to decide what you would want to do with all this information. Do you wish to switch from the regular diet to the Ketogenic diet? If your answer is yes then this book is your blueprint to getting your body in ketosis.

You should also be in a position to know that the book will not be accurate to the fullest which is why the book has recommended that you should seek the advice of your doctor or physician. You could learn more on the Ketogenic diet as new information keeps emerging given that this is not a thoroughly researched topic. The Ketogenic diet is still being studied on its abilities on different fronts.

It is also recommended to follow the diet that is recommended by your doctor or nutritionist and not simply what is offered in this book. Your doctor is better positioned to determine what your body desires and what is best for you. You could, however, use this book to enrich your knowledge of what to eat or what to avoid.

CPSIA information can be obtained
at www.ICGtesting.com
Printed in the USA
BVHW091406231120
593971BV00002B/520

9 781801 205931